Praise for *Ortho-Bionomy: A Path to Self-Care*

"It's portable Ortho-Bionomy for everyone! What could be better? Images, stories, and instruction provide a fabulous resource in reach of anyone seeking to increase physical comfort and expand that sense of being at home in oneself. In the simple spaciousness of Ortho-Bionomy self-care practice, we can tap into deep healing from within, a place where mind, body, and spirit are not separate. You won't need special equipment or clothing, only your time and this sublime and very practical compendium."

> —Christina Montes de Oca, advanced instructor and cofounder of the
> Ortho-Bionomy Practitioner Training Programs at the New Mexico
> Academy of Healing Arts

"This is a great collection of tools for patient self-care. Luann has been sharing these skills in her Ortho-Bionomy classes for over twenty-five years and now anyone can benefit from them by using this interactive book."

> —Pete Whitridge, LMT, massage instructor at the Florida School
> of Massage, Gainesville, Florida

"This book is a valuable resource for taking care of your body. The level of specificity makes it very practical for self-care."

> —Phillip Moffitt, director of the Life Balance Institute and author of
> *Dancing with Life: Buddhist Insights for Finding Meaning and Joy
> in the Face of Suffering*

"Ortho-Bionomy self-care exercises are a central part of my treatment of chronic pain patients. They are easy to perform and give people an immediate experience of their body's ability to improve. Ms. Overmyer brings a great depth and breadth of experience to the subject, both as a teacher and a lifelong student."

> —Kalpesh R. Patel, Ortho-Bionomy practitioner, Outpatient Physical
> Therapy Department, University of Florida Orthopaedics and Sports
> Medicine Institute

Ortho-Bionomy

A Path to Self-Care

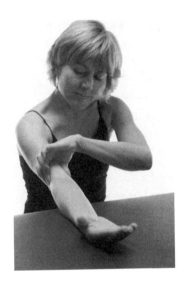

Simple
Techniques
to Release Pain
& Enhance
Well-Being

Luann Overmyer

North Atlantic Books
Berkeley, California

Published by
North Atlantic Books
P.O. Box 12327
Berkeley, California 94712

Cover photo by Denise Ritchie
Cover and book design by Jan Camp
Printed in the United States of America

Society of Ortho-Bionomy is a registered collective membership trademark of the Society of Ortho-Bionomy International, Inc., and used by the Society to indicate that a person using the mark is a member of the Society of Ortho-Bionomy and cannot be used without permission from the Society of Ortho-Bionomy International, Inc.

Ortho-Bionomy® is a trademark of the Society of Ortho-Bionomy International, Inc., and cannot be used without written permission from the Society of Ortho-Bionomy International, Inc.

Ortho-Bionomy: A Path to Self-Care is sponsored by the Society for the Study of Native Arts and Sciences, a nonprofit educational corporation whose goals are to develop an educational and cross-cultural perspective linking various scientific, social, and artistic fields; to nurture a holistic view of arts, sciences, humanities, and healing; and to publish and distribute literature on the relationship of mind, body, and nature.

North Atlantic Books' publications are available through most bookstores. For further information, visit our Web site at www.northatlanticbooks.com or call 800-733-3000.

Library of Congress Cataloging-in-Publication Data

Overmyer, Luann, 1948–
Ortho-Bionomy: a path to self-care / Luann Overmyer.
    p.; cm.
Includes bibliographical references and index.
Summary: "Presents positions, postures, and movements designed to release tension and ease pain. The techniques are simple to perform and can be done on one's own, without the use of special equipment. Positions for each part of the body are clearly described in lay terms and illustrated with photos and drawings"—Provided by publisher.
ISBN 978-1-55643-791-5
1. Osteopathic orthopedics. 2. Manipulation (Therapeutics) 3. Self-care, Health. I. Title.
[DNLM: 1. Manipulation, Orthopedic—methods. 2. Osteopathic Medicine. WB 535 O96o 2009]
RZ397.O94 2009
615.5'33—dc22

2009001462

2 3 4 5 6 7 8 9 SHERIDAN 15 14 13 12 11 10

Dedication

This book is dedicated to all those who seek relief from pain; to Arthur Lincoln Pauls who offered this simple method to everyone as an option for resolving pain; and to the practitioners and instructors of Ortho-Bionomy who apply skill, understanding, and compassion in aiding others to rediscover comfort within.

It is truly a pleasure to offer this book to you, the reader. May you discover for yourself the natural capacity within your body to relieve pain. May you enjoy a greater sense of comfort and well-being. And may these simple release techniques bring you to a greater awareness of your innate wholeness.

Acknowledgments

I wish to express my appreciation to all who have been teachers for me throughout the years: to Arthur Lincoln Pauls for developing the techniques of Ortho-Bionomy, to Gerda Alexander for her pioneering work in self-care, and particularly to my clients and students whose questions, conditions, and bodies have challenged me to deepen my understanding and question my assumptions.

I also wish to express my gratitude for the many osteopaths who have worked so gently with my body, repeatedly demonstrating to me the self-corrective reflexes at work within.

In retrospect, writing this book seems like the easy part. The challenge of crafting this book into a finished product was met with the skills and support of many people. I am grateful to Karen Casino for her hours of sustaining help with photographs. Our work together over the years helped me to develop a visual perspective for the book. Sara Sunstein's edits and organizational suggestions brought clarity and structure to the project. Lee Whitridge offered a discerning eye and practical advice. Denise Ritchie kept a cool head, a clear eye, and a steady hand during the photo shoots. Her professional yet easy-going nature kept the overwhelming task of shooting hundreds of photographs simple and straightforward. I am indebted to my photographic models Julie O'Neil, Stephanie Wild, Dick Frein, Mary Santello, Rima Zegarra, and Becky Waitz for their wellspring of good-natured presence and patience during the long hours of photo shoots. Jessica Sevey, my project editor at North Atlantic Books, guided this creative process with unflappable congeniality, clarity, and focused perspective.

Gratitude to the many who supported this project from the beginning and encouraged me through my learning curves: to Miranda Monkhorst and Brenda Sistrom who read, advised, and edited the early drafts; to Star Woodward and Pete Whitridge, my favorite on-call geeks, who assisted with computer skills as needed; to Carolyn Reynolds who made the illustrations seem easy. Loving appreciation to my family, friends, colleagues, and students for their faith and enthusiasm for this book.

MEDICAL DISCLAIMER: This book contains information and exercises to assist you to help yourself, to increase flexibility, and to relieve tension and pain. If you have doubts, or feel you cannot practice the exercises without pain, please consult a doctor or other qualified health practitioner. To find an Ortho-Bionomy practitioner or instructor in your area, please contact the Society of Ortho-Bionomy, International at www.ortho-bionomy.org.

Contents

FOREWORD

In those early formative years of the late 1970s and early 1980s, when I was studying with Arthur Lincoln Pauls, he made two things impeccably clear. First, he had a strong belief in what he called the "Evolvement of the Original Concept." As students we grappled with the question, "What is Ortho-Bionomy?" Arthur's interest was less in defining the work than expounding on the creative potential he saw inherent in the work. His teachings reflected the fluidity and plasticity available when applying the concepts of correcting through the laws of nature. He also had a strong desire to make this work available to everyone, regardless of degree, license, or previous experience. Because the simplicity of the concepts of Ortho-Bionomy make it possible to share the work with those from a myriad of backgrounds, it allows for incredible depth of response and practice.

And now the next generation of creative genius emerges regarding these original concepts. In the current publication Luann Overmyer has picked up these historic threads of Ortho-Bionomy and woven them into a remarkable resource for both practitioners and lay people alike. All readers will find this to be an imminently useful and ultimately practical guide to self-care and taking responsibility for one's health and well-being. Luann has taken Ortho-Bionomy to the next evolutionary spiral in the work as she continues to expand upon Arthur's original body of knowledge, as well as empower individuals in their quest for pain relief and restoring homeostasis of being.

Her years of experience in teaching and practicing Ortho-Bionomy come through the pages to reveal a masterwork of relevance in these times when assuming responsibility for one's own health takes on added significance. Could a comprehensive and easy-to-follow guide to pain management and self-care be of more value and timeliness, as 2009 opens us all to the profound new financial, political, and global realities that we face? Self-responsibility, empowerment, and caretaking of self and others are the missing elements necessary to restore balance in these tumultuous times. These themes run through the pages of this book, allowing people to take their well-being into their own hands. This is a book whose time has emerged in synchrony with changes of a more universal and planetary nature.

Luann has been teaching and expanding on the concepts of Self-Care in Ortho-Bionomy for many years. In a recent Self-Care class I was struck not only by her creativity in finding ways to support the body in the release positions but also her depth of experience in application. She was able to find ways to help individuals achieve positive results even in the face of profound pain and physical limitations. One consistent gift of Luann's is to never get lost in the student's or client's dysfunction. She has the capacity to stay strong and rely on her own circle of knowledge and her equally strong desire to help others. She generously shares this extensive knowledge base for the benefit of others in this publication. Ultimately Luann's goal is the desire for all individuals to experience the fullest and most expansive life possible, without hindrance of pain or other physical limitation. With this labor of love and life work before you she has taken one giant step forward toward reducing our collective suffering while allowing for the expansion of consciousness and true potentiality inherent in each and all of us.

—Denise Deig, MS, PT, GCFP, BFLT/T, Ortho-Bionomy instructor and author of *Positional Release Technique: From a Dynamic Systems Perspective*

PREFACE

The Accident

I was DOA, dead on arrival, according to the hospital staff.

Four hours earlier that warm summer evening in rural Indiana, July 1967, I'd been riding as passenger on my friend's motorcycle. As the bike flipped wheel-over-wheel down an embankment, I did too—my friend had been thrown off—and I found myself trapped beneath the heavy machine, handlebars wrapped around my neck.

My fear was intense, the injuries grave, yet after my friend dragged the cycle off me and climbed to the road to go for help, I found within myself a sense of calm witnessing. Taking inventory, I scanned my body with the clarity of the pre-med student that I was. I moved my legs. They seemed okay. My right arm couldn't move, and something was definitely wrong in my back. I noticed that I felt angry when I realized that I had surely broken some bones: my collarbone, some ribs, perhaps my spine. I noticed the sensations of the d̶___ ss and prickly weeds under the skin ___ s were serious and if I would die. I ___ for any transgressions that may have ___ lost consciousness.

___ ital after numerous detours, delays, ___ I was suddenly aware of seeing my ___ nd above the vehicle. Confused by ___ nt myself. From my position above ___ medical personnel who had come ___ inous, with brilliant light radiating

___ member asking myself, "Where am ___ d a transition in my consciousness, ___ uility and peacefulness.

The next thing I remember is seeing my body lying on a gurney at the side of the emergency room. "I" was up by the ceiling. The medical staff seemed occupied across the room. No one was attending to my body. As I tried to get someone's attention, I noticed a light surrounding one of the nurses. She asked me what I wanted.

"Why aren't you working on my body?" I inquired.

"If you want us to work on your body," she replied, "you must go back in."

"Oh, thank you … I didn't realize."

And so began my conscious journey into self-healing and self-care. I began to reinhabit my body at the rib cage, experiencing the density of matter and the slowness of molasses as I worked to reintegrate myself with my body. Body time seemed so, so slow compared to the quickness of my out-of-body perspective. Eventually I connected with my mind in a more familiar way and realized that I would now need to communicate with the hospital staff.

How do I get these people to notice that I am here? I wondered. I remembered movies where people were saved from being buried alive by wiggling their little finger. Unfortunately, my little finger was under the sheet. And then I had a memory of my mother saying, "The easiest thing to do is smile." I smiled and the staff noticed. Someone asked me why I was smiling. "I wanted you to know I was here."

A flurry of activity ensued as I was moved to the center of the room. This was a teaching hospital, and I would make excellent practice for the students since my prognosis was poor. Much to my dismay, they cut off my clothes. I had sewn that outfit myself! An incision was made in my ankle. When I protested that nothing was wrong with my ankle, I was informed that it was for the intravenous solution.

"Hmm … it's not going to work … I have poor circulation in my feet."

"Trust us; we know what we are doing."

Some time later they realized that it wasn't working and made another incision in my femoral artery. Calmly, I watched as a new intern attempted to make a cut in my upper chest to place a tube into my collapsed lung. The supervising doctor said she hadn't gone deep enough and made the cut himself. I seemed to be distant from the whole process, but at least I was no longer on the ceiling.

Investigative surgery was hours long, with students practicing their skills under supervision. It was early morning when my body arrived in the intensive care unit. With severe injuries and four hours without adequate medical attention, my chances of survival were fifty-fifty. I had a broken clavicle and ribs, a punctured and collapsed lung, internal bleeding caused by a torn hepatic ligament and a lacerated liver, and a spine fractured in three places (which wasn't discovered until five days later). Every two hours family members could visit for fifteen minutes. I remember awakening for some of those visits, my internal mood perky, my body slow to express.

On the fourth day, I was moved into a sitting position to allow my lungs some exercise. Although I protested that the pain in my back was intense, the nurses insisted and handed me a hairbrush. I felt overwhelmed with pain and wept. The next morning I complained bitterly about my back pain to the doctor checking my abdominal sutures. More x-rays were ordered, taken with me sitting up instead of lying down. Doctors were surprised to find that, indeed, I had compressed fractures in three thoracic vertebrae. Now it was decided that I shouldn't be sitting, and the residents questioned my capacity to even move my legs, feet, and toes. An orthopedic back brace was ordered.

The day I was transferred from intensive care to a regular ward was an emotional one. All day tears fell with realizations of how I had escaped death and questions of why I had survived. Repeatedly I asked myself, "If I'm here, what is it that I'm supposed to do?"

The poetic response was always the same: "It doesn't matter what; it matters that the how is whole." At the time I didn't know what this meant, but the words made a strong impact on me, staying with me to this day.

Once the brace arrived, I was promised that I could go home as soon as I could walk. Thus motivated, I got moving and was released in a few days.

About a week later, at my next checkup with the orthopedic doctor, I was told that my body was too bent over and that I needed to practice walking in front of a mirror. "If you don't straighten up, you will have to wear a full body cast for a year," he threatened. I stood in front of the mirror and tried to arrange my internal sensations to match the desired external reflection. With practice I gained a more upright posture.

I returned to UCLA that fall and threw myself into campus life, kept busy, and did my best to ignore the discomfort and inconvenience of my injuries and healing process. Yet my near-death experience had touched me, and I felt the need to explore, experience, and understand myself in as whole a way as possible. I changed my major from pre-med to psychology and education.

My Early Explorations in Ortho-Bionomy®

A few years later, my discomfort became impossible to ignore, and my self-healing journey was pushed to another level. Trying chiropractic, I appreciated that I felt better for a few hours after treatments, and I reasoned that pain-free alignment was possible. I just needed to learn how to maintain the alignment for longer than a few hours. By now I was living in the Bay Area in Northern California, and I decided to explore my options. I enrolled in classes in massage, bodywork, movement awareness, and meditation. I learned to quiet my mind, sense my body directly, and increase my awareness of comfort and alignment. My studies with a renowned physiotherapist improved my understanding of anatomy, and I gained skills for working with others.

Around this same time, I hurt my neck during a hiking accident. Since my chiropractor had moved away, I decided to see the chiropractor a friend suggested.

This chiropractor examined my swollen neck with gentle palpation and diagnosed a serious whiplash. He barely touched my neck, and all of a sudden I was experiencing myself in many different ways: physically, emotionally, mentally, psychologically, energetically, kinesthetically, and spiritually. Each way was familiar, yet the overall experience was completely surprising to me. Intrigued, I asked what he was doing. This was not like any chiropractic treatment I had ever received. He told me that this method was called Ortho-Bionomy. He had learned it from a British osteopath named Arthur Lincoln Pauls.

This gentle, non-intrusive contact evoked within me such a strong, clear, and personal experience of myself, and gently and effectively released my pain at the same time. Fascinated, I knew I had to investigate this method further and asked about classes. I learned that Arthur Lincoln Pauls, who developed this work, would be returning to San Francisco in six months, and anyone could take the course.

I set my focus during the first class to learn how to release my own neck. Even though I had a massage practice by now, I was more interested in seeing if this work would be effective for me before I began to apply it with others. The techniques were relatively simple, and I felt supported in the learning process. As the class continued, I was impressed by the ease with which tension and pain could be released. No thrust techniques, no intense probings, essentially no pain or discomfort at all. Just gentle, specific positioning that actually released tension and relieved pain fast. My neck felt much better by the end of class. My sense of chronic tension, lumpy tightness, and discomfort was replaced with more range of motion, ease of movement, and a feeling of well-being.

The following week, I continued to work with my neck whenever I felt tension or pain. I discovered that I could even find the release position while driving. When I maintained this position for a minute or so, tension actually discharged, the lumpiness dissipated, and the pain disappeared. I felt hooked on this stuff.

Not only was I learning skills for self-care and helping my massage clients, I gained understanding about my own healing process from something Pauls had said: "An organism can only accept so much change at a time. During a session you may experience some tension release. Then as the body integrates that change, more release may continue to occur."

This was very true in my case. Over time, as my neck continued to release, it slowly began to return toward alignment at a pace that could be supported. I realized then that my neck had not been able to support the alignment techniques of the first chiropractor because the change had been too rapid. My neck muscles needed a slower process than adjustments to understand how to release the tension pattern on their own, and they also needed time to develop the strength to support new alignment. I recognized how the Ortho-Bionomy work respected the natural healing pace of the body.

It was explained that at the moment of an accident the muscles tighten in an attempt to protect the body, yet these protective tension patterns can remain long after they are useful. The body integrates the patterns and sees them as important and so continues to repeat the protective pattern of tension—just like what happens in a whiplash injury when the neck muscles tighten so the neck does not break. Yet the whiplash tension pattern prevails and the neck loses its capacity for normal range of movement and function. By gently and slowly allowing the neck to relax, the body can integrate the release and remember to return to its natural alignment. Factoring the muscles into the equation of alignment made sense to me, and my personal experience with the slower and gentler release techniques of Ortho-Bionomy gave me longer-lasting relief.

Soon after the first class I began to include the techniques and apply the principles of Ortho-Bionomy in my practice of therapeutic massage. I appreciated how easy the techniques were to use, and how I could get better results with less work on my part. I watched my clients release their pain, increase their range of motion, and recover their functionality. Clients reported amazement as their symptoms disappeared. They said they felt lighter, more relaxed, and more at ease in their daily lives. One client who was suffering from intense pain after ankle surgery called to express her gratitude and to tell me that all her pain was gone after only one session.

Then a friend brought her boyfriend for a session. He had been born with spasticity. The muscles in his lower back and pelvis were tightly locked up and twisted to almost a ninety-degree angle. The spasms also shortened his muscles, causing him to limp. He was very motivated to change his body and posture. He had gone through Rolfing twice but still had severe patterns of spasm. I was just a beginner and felt a bit overwhelmed tackling such a case, but I thought about the principles of self-correction and decided that it wouldn't hurt to try. Simply move the body toward ease, and support the position of comfort. Add slight compression so the muscles shorten and the body releases its holding patterns and returns to balance. Allow the body to pace its own healing.

After his first session I explained to him that, according to my teacher, the work would continue even after the session. This was convenient since he lived more than six hundred miles away, making frequent treatments unlikely. Three months after the session, he called to ask me how long the releasing was going to continue, because he wanted to buy new pants. He said that since the session with me his leg had steadily continued to lengthen and his pants were not long enough now, but he didn't want to go out and spend money on new pants yet if his leg length was going to continue to change. I was honestly shocked to hear that anything had happened at all. Over the next couple of years I worked with him only twice more, and each time his leg would begin a new phase of lengthening as his spasms continued to release.

About five years after our initial session, I visited him and my friend, now living in Europe. He asked if I wanted to see the difference in his spine and removed his shirt. The change was amazing. His spine had completely straightened out, and his pelvis had unlocked all the muscle spasms. I wouldn't have believed it possible. When he asked for my reaction, I congratulated him on his good work.

I told him that I felt drawn to work with his feet and perhaps release his psoas muscle. Surprisingly, he responded that he had never had any problems with his feet until the last few months, but now they were bothering him all the time. So I worked with the positioning techniques for his feet and his psoas muscle. The next morning, he came to breakfast smiling, saying that this was the first time in months that his feet didn't hurt and his shoes felt comfortable.

As I thought about this progression of symptoms, I remembered that Arthur Pauls had talked about Ortho-Bionomy following the principles of homeopathy: healing would occur from the top of the body down, from the present back through past injuries, and from the inside to the outside. This certainly seemed to pertain to my friend's case: as his back and pelvis cleared, the pattern moved down and out to his feet.

Ortho-Bionomy: The How Is Whole

As I practiced Ortho-Bionomy, it became obvious to me that this work was much more effective for my clients than anything else I had learned. Tight, tense shoulder muscles could release in seconds without my having to strain my thumbs with deep-tissue massage techniques. Clients were mystified that such gentle contact and positioning could give such quick relief from tension and pain. As people began requesting more Ortho-Bionomy and less massage, my skills for facilitating the body's self-corrective reflexes increased. I learned to sense and understand underlying patterns of holding within the body—for example, connections between shoulder tension and lack of support in the low back; the relationship between posture and spinal flexibility and structural stability; and the importance of balanced tone for health and well-being.

More importantly, though, my respect for the natural self-corrective reflexes of the body grew. My hands listened to the body, and my mind and my heart listened, too. While my clients began to notice an increasing sense of comfort and ease within their bodies, I began noticing that their worry and complaints about their lives diminished. It seemed that the physical sense of relaxation carried over to other aspects of their lives, helping them release emotional and mental uneasiness and reduce their anxieties. As they expanded their range of motion, their capacity for more effectively managing the difficult aspects of their life also grew. They learned to trust themselves more and to trust the inherent wisdom within, and I learned to trust and respect the process of the natural self-corrective capacity of the individual.

Yet something else was happening with clients as well.

I remember asking one of my early and most regular clients if he would be willing to make a statement about the work for a brochure I was putting together. Tom was a truck driver who worked out with weights, and I thought of him as a very physically oriented person. He responded that he wouldn't know what to say because each session was a spiritual experience for him.

Upon reflection, I realized the truth within his statement. I thought back to my early experiences of Ortho-Bionomy with the first practitioner, to my amazement over how the work gently offered me an experience of my wholeness through my body. I remembered the sensations of my first session and the clear perspective of myself as a physical, emotional, mental, energetic, and spiritual being. I thought back to my hospital experience after the accident, to the light from the nurse who communicated to me to go back into my body, and to my question to myself concerning what I was meant to do since I hadn't died. The answer that had come had seemed poetic to me at the time, but it made sense for me now. "It doesn't matter what, it matters that the how is whole."

Ortho-Bionomy is certainly the most whole modality of any that I have studied. At its center is respect for the individual at all levels of being. My practice of Ortho-Bionomy has confirmed for me the wondrous effects of approaching the individual as a living whole: body, mind, emotions, energy, soul, spirit.

So I welcome you to this exploration of your own wholeness as you focus on your body's ability to return to ease.

Thirty Years Later

My psychology studies prepared me to work with people, to be curious and compassionate, to observe the emotions, and to trust the process. Through the practice of meditation I have learned to slow down, observe my own mind and body, and to be compassionate in my work with others. For me, Ortho-Bionomy began as a way to self-heal. It stimulated my curiosity in the body and offered a path for assisting others to find comfort and ease. Thirty years of private practice have taught me to honor the inherent wisdom of the body, to appreciate the unique ways that healing and self-recognition can take place, and to have faith in the amazing resources of the body/mind for self-healing.

I continued my studies with the founder of Ortho-Bionomy, British osteopath Arthur Lincoln Pauls, until his death in 1997. In the late '80s I had the opportunity to study with Gerda Alexander from Copenhagen, the founder of Eutony. Her influence renewed and rekindled my interest in Self-Care. I felt inspired to develop specific, teachable Ortho-Bionomy Self-Care techniques and began to incorporate them into my private practice and trainings.

Ortho-Bionomy lends itself perfectly to self-care in both concept and reality. Teaching others to tune into the body, to be present with what is, and to recognize the natural capacity for gentle self-regulation for pain relief and increased well-being is a wonderful way to make a living. And I haven't been bored yet. I enjoy witnessing the increased empowerment and delight as each person discovers the ability to attune to comfort and effect genuine pain relief by applying the principles and techniques of Ortho-Bionomy Self-Care. I appreciate how much this work empowers individuals to discover their own resources for pain relief, comfort, and well-being.

Teaching throughout the United States and Australia, I see that Ortho-Bionomy is always well-received and embraced by hands-on professionals looking for more tools, as well as by regular folks looking for a way to help themselves, their family, and friends. I can't tell you how many times I have heard people say that they feel they have come home to themselves with this work. And I know that a crucial part of my keeping healthy with such a busy lifestyle is my being able to practice Ortho-Bionomy Self-Care exercises to release pain as it arises and to reestablish comfort from within.

INTRODUCTION

Is This Book for You?

This book provides a step-by-step guide to help you release tensions and pain throughout your body, while also increasing your ability to feel and create comfort and relaxation. Whether you feel stress at the end of the day, pain from an injury or chronic condition, or want to enhance wellness, Ortho-Bionomy Self-Care supports your goal. Using safe, comfortable positioning and gentle movement exercises, you will come to recognize and engage the resources within your own body that allow you to heal and feel better rapidly.

Regardless of age or physical condition, everyone can benefit from Ortho-Bionomy Self-Care. No special clothing, equipment, or regimen is required, simply your time, attention, and a willingness to feel better and learn something new.

With Ortho-Bionomy Self-Care you can release back pain, neck pain, tight shoulders, and rib pain. You can find relief for ankle sprains, foot and knee pain, arthritic pain, tension headaches, sciatica, and scoliosis. You can learn gentle ways of addressing the discomfort and tension patterns that contribute to fibromyalgia, repetitive strain, and arm pain. Every technique in this book can lead to greater ease and improved well-being.

Because Ortho-Bionomy is fundamentally about the inherent capacity of the individual to self-correct, it naturally lends itself to self-care techniques. It makes sense to teach people to attune to this self-healing process and to empower them to use the simple techniques for pain and tension relief. Arthur Pauls, the British osteopath who developed Ortho-Bionomy, often talked about the importance of giving students exercises at the end of sessions so they could continue reminding the body of its natural ability to release and self-correct.

One client taught me about this. She came for regular sessions and would engage in casual conversation about various topics, all completely unrelated to what we were doing. Although my sense was that this didn't support her releasing at a deeper level, conversation seemed to make her more comfortable than relaxing into her body. Then one day she arrived to say, much to my surprise, that she had tried many of the positions at home to successfully release tension in her spine. After this experience I began to actively include self-care exercises into the sessions.

I gradually learned to modify the positional techniques for self-care and to assist clients in attuning to their own internal sense of comfort and capacity. Adapting the techniques for self-care in my own body and for my clients gradually led me to develop a class of Self-Care exercises and to write this book.

With thirty years in private practice and teaching Ortho-Bionomy Self-Care seminars, I am convinced that people are motivated, capable, and willing to work with themselves to relieve pain when they have the information and tools to do so.

When to practice self-care:

Each exercise suggests how long and how often to practice. A general guideline is to set aside a daily time to tune into yourself and truly attend to your body's sensations and healing process. The amount of time is sometimes less important than the quality of time. Most individual positions and exercises take about ten minutes, and you may want to do several in a row to address tensions in adjacent areas.

What you will need:

Warm floor space (carpeted or use a folded blanket)

- Chair, couch, or bed
- Pillows
- Folded hand towels
- Soft hollow rubber ball—I particularly like Gertie Balls (available at www.smallworldtoys.com)
- Two tennis balls in a sock

The Doctor Inside

Genuine healing comes from within. When we slow down and listen to our body's responses, we are trusting and we thereby affirm and assist our recuperative potential. We also engage our inner wisdom in support of self-healing.

As we mature, though, we can become conditioned to believe that others know more than we do about the workings of our body. If we have pain or feel out of sorts, then the doctor, nutritionist, herbalist, homeopath, acupuncturist, psychologist, or some other "expert" will know what to do. Although these professionals may certainly have information that could be useful to us, it is important not to override one's own sense of what feels right. An overdependence on outside experts or authorities shifts the focus away from sensing our own experience and discovering within ourselves the inherent possibility for self-soothing.

Such transference away from our inner authority to an outer authority gradually creates a mistrust of our inherent potential. We lose connection with our inner knowing and become further dependent on others to "heal" us. And when "healing" comes in the form of drugs, we further confuse our sensory capacities to self-regulate.

When my daughter was three years old she cut her thumb, and she came to me crying and confused. The thumb continued to bleed even as we applied pressure. As I comforted her, I realized my inadequacy in determining if she needed stitches. I thought about a trip to the hospital emergency room, a likely long wait, and perhaps a needless expense. I wondered if it was really necessary. I knew the body heals itself, yet this was my injured daughter, and I wanted to do the best thing for her well-being. I looked at the cut once more and then said to her, "There is a doctor inside you who knows exactly what you need to do. Why don't you close your eyes and ask what you should do?"

She closed her eyes, was still for a moment, and then announced, "I need to take a nap now" and proceeded to go to her room and fall asleep. After her nap the cut had closed, the bleeding stopped, and she no longer felt pain or discomfort. The cut healed up perfectly without a trace.

When I was a child, I asked questions about the smallest symptoms. How does a splinter work its way out all by itself? Why does a bruise turn purple? And then yellow? And then how does the skin eventually become normal again? Some responses carried a warning: "Don't scratch that chicken pox. It will leave a scar." *What is a scar?* I wondered.

Once, my big toe got caught in a car door. Pain aside, I was very upset about my toe. What would happen to it now? When I was told that the toenail would get black and fall off and then a new one would grow, I was sad and scared. I didn't want any part of me to get black and fall off, so I decided that it wasn't going to happen to me that way. Imagine my delight when, in fact, the toenail healed perfectly without getting black or falling off. This incident reinforced my childish "magical thinking." I still wonder about the role my decision played in not losing the toenail. Did it reconnect me with the doctor within?

Magical thinking has matured and gained popularity and credibility in the form of visualization exercises. In clinical practice, I've repeatedly found that visualization of an attempted movement increases the ability to move. Visualizing an outcome cues and empowers the nervous system to increase movement potential.

George, a gentleman in his sixties, had suffered a stroke six years prior. The range of motion and use of his left arm was limited. His left elbow was bent and appeared glued to his side, and his left hand was held tightly across his waist. Without trying to move his arm at all, I lightly contacted one of the shoulder release points and then gently compressed from the elbow toward the shoulder joint. I slowly worked through each of the eight shoulder points and added compression from the elbow each time. Then I focused on his right arm, moving it into specific release positions. I suggested to George that he visualize his left arm moving into these same positions that I was creating with the right arm.

After a few minutes, he began to move his left arm. Compression and visualization had awakened his reflexive movement potential. As yet he couldn't control the movement very specifically, due to the disturbed nerve circuits caused by his stroke, but the reflex potential was indeed working. It would be available now to help him build new connections and increase his movement capacity.

The qualities of curiosity, magical thinking, and inner authority are essential elements in our own self-care. Curiosity helps us to focus our attention and brings us to an awareness of what is really happening. What do we sense? What makes it change? What makes it feel better? Magical thinking gathers our wonderment and exercises our playful will to not be satisfied with predictable outcomes. If we can imagine a different outcome, perhaps we can physically create one. And our inner authority enables us to trust the doctor within. It supports our innate ability to self-regulate and heal.

What's Stress Got to Do with It?

Pain and discomfort can bring up many emotional responses: panic, fear, uncertainty, confusion, impatience, anger, sadness, depression. Our thinking mind may validate these feelings, but it can also amplify them.

Say you awaken to feel your lower back locked up. There is pain and weakness when you try to stand, and you worry about how you'll get through the day. Then confusion sets in about how to deal with the situation. Perhaps you feel anger about not being able to carry out your scheduled activities or meet your obligations.

One's mind can leap to fears of worst possible scenarios: surgery, paralysis, disability. We may panic about how we will continue to make a living, or be able to pay for the care we need. Each of these emotions and feeling states can seem valid to our thinking mind.

But revving our emotions doesn't decrease the pain, and it often increases the stress, puts nerves on edge, and doesn't do much to help the body. How can we access our natural self-balancing reflexes in stressful situations? We could take a cue from my young daughter who somehow knew within herself that taking a nap would help her calm down, slow the blood flow, and allow the body to heal.

Sometimes the demands of life seem to come at us with such speed. If we continuously try to keep pace with the speed, we can create a condition of permanent stress for ourselves. Our system gets "stuck" in hyper-drive, with our nerves attempting to respond to every situation that comes up. This fatigues the body's calming system and ability to maintain internal balance. After a while we become chronically tired, unable to get enough rest, and our functioning suffers. We no longer can get to deep restful states for replenishment, rejuvenation, and well-being. This imbalance cannot go on continually without affecting the balanced functioning of our organ systems and our ability to heal.

Becoming conscious of our nervous system's revving and calming responses is another step toward self-care. Calm restfulness is crucial for releasing pain and tension and also for the overall health and vitality of mind and body.

THE STRESS RESPONSE

The autonomic nervous system supports and controls our survival and vital functioning automatically, without our consciously thinking about it. It has two parts, the sympathetic and parasympathetic.

Sympathetic: The sympathetic nervous system readies the body to respond automatically to danger, stress, and emotional states. In preparing the body to spring into action, it increases blood flow to the muscles and raises the heart rate and blood pressure. In situations of perceived danger, it signals the adrenaline response necessary to give us the energy to move quickly. All that is involved in our "readiness response" comes under the effects of the sympathetic nervous system.

Parasympathetic: The parasympathetic nervous system oversees the functioning of vital organs and glands and assists long-range vitality. It is restorative and nurturing to our viscera and functions best during rest and sleep states. The parasympathetic nervous system increases blood flow to the organs and lowers heart rate and blood pressure. It facilitates digestion and assimilation of food, and fosters elimination. As a part of its functions, the parasympathetic system counteracts and balances the action-oriented fight-or-flight reflex of the sympathetic system. It is good to remember that the parasympathetic system has its own deeper, vitalizing work to do during quiet restful periods.

Accessing the Calm Witness

The first steps to creating nervous system balance involve learning to detect your own signs of imbalance. Notice your breath, notice the pace of respiration, notice any tensions in your body, and notice your emotional responses to various stimuli. With awareness, we can learn ways to reduce the evidence of stress within us and assist our restorative and recuperative capacity.

There is a mood or quality to practicing Ortho-Bionomy Self-Care that includes calm witnessing. This relaxed yet attentive state allows the experience to be observed just as it is. We suspend the chatter of a judging mind that can so often lead to anxiety, worry, and fear. By placing one's mind in neutral, the body has the opportunity to communicate direct experience. This gives the nervous system and the rest of the body the opportunity to recalibrate and self-correct. Within this state of calm witnessing, worries and anxiety about the body and pain are suspended.

SQUARE BREATHING

This breathing technique called "Square Breathing" from Pranayama yoga can be used to balance and relax the nervous system so we can be present within ourselves without anxiety or worry. Regulating the breath brings a sense of balanced rhythm to the nervous system. The calm, quiet witness emerges from within this relaxed state. Emotions calm down, the thinking mind quiets, and the body's reflexive nature can access its self-correcting capacity.

1. Begin by inhaling as you count to four.

2. Hold the inhalation for another count of four.

3. Exhale for a count of four.

4. Hold the exhalation for a count of four.

I visualize drawing each side of a square as I count: as I breathe in and count to four, I draw one wall of the square. As I hold my breath for another count of four, I draw the top of the square. As I exhale to a count of four, I visualize drawing the wall parallel to the first side. As I hold the exhalation for the final count, I draw the bottom of the square. Then I begin again and retrace my square.

If at first this seems too difficult, try drawing a rectangle instead. Breathe in to a count of four, hold for a count of two, exhale to a count of four, and hold for a count of two. As you become more accustomed to regulating your breathing pattern, it will get easier to draw and breathe a square.

※ ※ ※

It is essential to have alertness, curiosity, and calm to investigate your experience as you work with yourself. Focusing on your physical sensation connects your awareness to your bodily experience.

Necessity drives many individuals to pay attention to their body. An injury that causes limitation or pain is a great motivator to figure out what works, what feels comfortable and what doesn't. Without attention to your body's responses, the body's range of movement may become limited, and the mind can become stuck in thinking that the limitation is all that is possible.

Bringing awareness to your body as you practice these exercises and release techniques helps you to differentiate which positions and exercises bring the best relief. As you come into an interested, working relationship with your body, your awareness, understanding, and appreciation of your self-regulating capacity for well-being will grow, as will your ability to find comfort easily and naturally.

Discover and Cultivate the Attitude of Comfort

Our attitudes toward pain can take us out of ourselves, creating such a feeling of dissociation that our quality of life is impacted. The irritation of the pain colors every experience. When pain becomes the only thing we feel, we lose touch with joy or serenity and become irritated with all of life. We lose our capacity to differentiate various sensations.

I have heard it said that much of our pain is a learned response to an initial painful stimulus. We begin to tighten or contract in response to the pain, and soon we begin to contract in anticipation of it, slowly and gradually decreasing our natural range of motion. We grow accustomed to noticing it and to checking in to see if it is still there, or tensing to protect ourselves from the possibility of feeling it. Pain seems to become so familiar to our daily life that we cannot imagine being without it.

What would happen, however, if we began to notice and focus on sensations of comfort with the same degree of attention that we have put toward pain? Perhaps comfort can be learned as well. Perhaps we could begin to observe and alert ourselves to ease just by noticing what feels better. As we sense what feels better, we could move toward it. The more frequently we move toward what makes us feel good, the more we come to anticipate relief. By noticing and responding to our preferences for ease, we gradually learn to substitute a painful habit with a more comfortable one. Practicing Ortho-Bionomy Self-Care can be as simple as that.

When we slow down and begin to notice and track our sensations, we begin to discover which movements promote comfort and ease, and we start to recognize that there are differences, even if subtle. Small amounts of ease can begin to replace overwhelming pain. With care and attention to being gentle with ourselves, we learn to tune into our physical sensations without the familiar attitude of painful expectation. Gradually we begin to recognize that we have a choice each moment to notice what feels better and move toward it. This awareness and attunement to our sensation empowers us in the process of self-healing and moves us closer to the embodiment of well-being.

Memorizing the Sensations of Comfort

Once you recognize the sensations of relaxation, you can practice returning to those sensations and that mood. Imagine yourself relaxing: notice the body softening and allow yourself to savor the sensations. Then anchor it in your mental and body memory. When clients report feeling much more comfortable in themselves after a session, I tell them to memorize the feeling and evoke it when they need to remind themselves of ease. In this same way, we begin the process of reeducating ourselves to return to comfort.

How Does Ortho-Bionomy Positioning Work?

In my first Ortho-Bionomy class, Arthur Pauls talked about the self-corrective reflexes of the body. From his Judo training, he had recognized the body's reflexive ability to regain and maintain balance quickly. He explained this with Newton's Third Law of Motion: For every action there is an opposite and equal reaction, and for every interaction there is a pair of forces at work.

From his osteopathic practice, Pauls understood that a natural range of motion is the balanced effect of opposing muscles around the joint. Working in pairs, muscles on one side of the joint stretch and lengthen while the muscles on the opposite side contract and shorten. If one muscle group becomes over-contracted and can't respond to internal prompts, then the opposing muscle or group of muscles remains chronically overstretched. When the body holds on to such an unbalanced pairing, ease and normal range of movement are compromised.

Often, in an attempt to avoid pain, the body constricts and contracts surrounding muscles to prevent movement. Fear of pain reinforces the holding. Immobilization may solve the pain problem in the moment, but it can set up compensatory tension and holding patterns that limit healing and subsequent reestablishment of normal movement.

Pauls theorized that if you remind the body of what it is doing—in other words, if you slightly overstretch the overstretched muscle and slightly compress the contracted muscle—then the body recognizes and self-corrects.

While part of this self-recognition comes from the muscles' amount of stretch, nerves for proprioception play a big part as well. Proprioceptive nerves inform the body about its position and regulate positioning and movement. They are stimulated by movement and compression.

Of course this was all good in theory, but how could it be applied?

Pauls's opportunity came during a session with a woman whose cervical spine was so locked up that he couldn't move her neck into any position without causing intense pain. Noting the direction of the muscle tension pattern, he supported her neck in the contracted position, and he ever so slightly brought the neck joints closer together, further shortening the muscles. Suddenly the woman's neck began moving all by itself and released all its tension and pain.

By supporting her most comfortable position, which was approximately how she was already holding herself, Pauls had tapped into the body's reflexive capacity to instinctively self-correct, to release tensions and reestablish ease and normal range of motion. Just like a knot in a shoelace, if you take up the slack and push toward the knot, it will unravel more easily. Or a window that gets stuck—sometimes if you push it closed first, you will find it is easier to open.

I. Preparation

CHAPTER 1

Getting Started:
What You Need to Know

Using the Self-Care Section

The Self-Care Techniques are structured in a functional presentation that makes sense for most of my students, and ideally for you, too. Each technique builds on previous ones in terms of both structural integrity and written information. Many descriptions begin with pithy tidbits and anecdotes gleaned from my years of practice and study. They have implications broader than that specific body part, so you'll want to be sure to read them, even if you don't feel a need for that particular technique.

We begin with the low back (lumbar spine) and pelvis, which are the literal foundation for healthy posture. The hips, legs, and feet, connecting us with the earth, complete the foundational picture. The techniques then return to the spine—the mid and upper back (thoracic spine). After you release the upper and lower back, techniques for posture are possible. The rib cage, shoulders, arms, and hands follow. The neck and head, including the eyes, ears, and jaw, round out our treatment of the body. The last section covers Special Conditions such as cumulative stress disorders associated with postural dysfunction, scoliosis, sciatica, and bunions.

Despite the aforementioned, feel free to skip through this book, using the releases and exercises that address your particular problem.

The body is a living, working organism with interdependent systems, so you may need to address neighboring and/or related parts to complete a release and to restore ease and functionality. Get to know the neighborhoods and promote friendly relationships.

Before attempting any exercise or release, make sure that you have read through the directions completely and understand the sequence of movements. It's most helpful if you can visualize and even sense yourself doing the position or exercise before you move through the physical actuality.

It is more important that you discover and use what works for you than follow any protocols I may suggest. Remember that these exercises are intended to assist you in finding comfort and ease for yourself, not as a substitute for medical attention.

Types of Self-Care Exercises

- **For pain relief and to release tension,** use the Release Positions.
- **To maintain mobility and flexibility,** use the Movement exercises.
- **For quick releases,** use Isometric and Isotonic exercises.
- **To cue the body to potential movement capacity,** and for strengthening new patterns, use Isometric and Isotonic exercises.
- **To explore more deeply your movement patterning,** use the Awareness exercises.

Release Positioning techniques release muscular tension patterns. They interrupt compensation and holding patterns established at the time of injury and help to reset the natural self-corrective reflexes.

Breathing exercises increase oxygenation of tissues and stimulate relaxation, increasing the capacity to heal. Relaxed use of the breath creates a sense of internal massage, reestablishing a natural calming rhythm within.

Movement exercises release tension patterns, and cue the proprioceptive nervous system to recognize a wider range of functional options. Movement is critical for learning, and it can generate new neural pathways.

Awareness exercises focus the attention on the experience of directly sensing the body. This act of sensing with awareness brings insight and trust and increases function and comfort. Muscles organize for movement based on where the initiation of movement occurs. Awareness assists the potential for reeducation.

Isometric and Isotonic exercises (described below) assist in releasing muscle tension patterns, awaken the nervous system to specific movement potential, and increase strength and range of movement capacity.

Visualization of the attempted movement before and/or during the process enhances the results, especially of isometrics and isotonics. Inviting the brain and nervous system to attune to another way, visualization helps to release limiting patterns of hesitation, fear, or restriction of movement potential.

Isometric and Isotonic Movements: An Explanation

Isometric and isotonic exercises are useful when an injury such as a frozen shoulder limits range of movement. They are also beneficial when fear of pain causes the nervous system to limit range of motion.

"Iso" means "same." *Isometric* means "same length." In an *isometric* exercise, gentle movement using only about 20% of your strength is attempted and met with an equal resistance that prevents movement. This resistance to attempted movement is held for seven to ten seconds and then released to allow the attempted motion to be completed and to sense the increased movement potential.

In this way, the muscle is held at one length even though the nervous system is attempting to signal the muscle to lengthen. An isometric exercise can release an over-shortened muscle or help reset the cueing mechanism. This interrupts holding and tension patterns and reminds the body of its potential.

Isotonic means "same tone." In an *isotonic* exercise, gentle resistance is applied against movement but, rather than stopping movement, it permits slow, even movement, so the muscle works through its range of motion while maintaining a steady tone or force (once again about 20%). An isotonic exercise tones and strengthens a muscle through its entire range of motion.

During an isometric exercise, resistance allows no movement. During an isotonic exercise, slow, steady movement is allowed against resistance.

In Ortho-Bionomy all isometric and isotonic exercises begin from a position of comfort; then light resistance, about a half pound, is applied as you attempt to move out of the position with 20% strength. After ten seconds, the body part is moved passively to follow though the attempted movement in order to reinforce the increased range. Often the two are used in tandem, beginning with an isometric to engage the muscle and followed with an isotonic to affirm and strengthen the range of motion. It is important to remember to support the follow-through movement after resistance in both isometric and isotonic exercises.

Points and Positions of Release

About Release Positions

1. Every painful or tender point or area of the body has a position that will relieve the pain.

2. Facilitating a release depends on finding just the right position for *your* body.

3. Finding the best position for your body requires calm, curiosity, exploration, and non-judging attention.

4. Move in and out of the positioning slowly and gently to avoid rushing past the "just-right" place. Slow down and explore.

5. The position of release closely approximates the way the body is already holding. For example, if one of your shoulders is higher than the other, the position may be one that takes that shoulder higher to create comfort.

6. Generally the position of release "curls," "caves," or "folds" around the tender point/area and softens the area of tension and relieves the pain.

7. If you are in the correct position the indicator point will no longer be sore. If the point is somewhat less tender, it means you are in the

ballpark. That position may work or you may need to fine-tune the positioning for a more complete release of the tension pattern.

8. Slight compression toward the joint helps the body to recognize the imbalance and stimulates a self-correcting reflex, so compression is included in most of the positions.

9. You may sense release in many different ways:

    • Increased sense of comfort and relief

    • Spontaneous deep breath

    • Gradual relaxation

    • Gurgling in your abdomen

    • Softening or a light pulsation at the formerly tense point or area

    • Buzzing or aching sensation in your monitoring finger

10. Be sure to move out of the positioning slowly so as not to restimulate the dysfunctional pattern that you have just released.

11. After a release, be gentle with yourself. Avoid the temptation to check the area by moving in ways that might restimulate the tension pattern. Give the releases time to integrate naturally. Remember, the body is still healing even after the pain is gone: help foster that healing by being mindful to not overdo.

12. If tension returns, take time to go back into the release position to gently remind the body of comfort.

Indicator Points

Any tender point in the body can be used as an indicator point, and there are also specific indicator points that we use. Also referred to as *tension points, release points,* or *reflex points,* indicator points help you to assess strain, tension, and pain. Often they are referred tension originating from a different location. For example, we use indicator points on the front of the pelvis to identify imbalances in the low back and pelvis.

Generally, release occurs by caving or folding the area around the point. Each indicator point is matched with a specific position to release tension and pain. If you assess the point during positioning and sense no tension or tenderness, you'll know you are in the optimal position. After the positioning, you may recheck the indicator points to see if pain or discomfort has lessened or completely cleared there. Try the suggested position or use one that you discover feels more comfortable.

Making a light contact with the pad of the middle finger helps direct the body's focus during positioning and release. This is referred to as "monitoring" the point, because we are observing subtle changes through the fingertip. You may feel the tissue soften or feel heat or pulsation in your monitoring finger. You may also feel a buzzing, or a cramping or achy sensation. This sometimes happens as the body discharges excess energy from the point. If this happens it may help to raise the index finger off the body while continuing to monitor with the middle finger.

II. Foundation and Ground—
Lower Body

⫿ ⫿ ⫿

CHAPTER 2

Low Back

Finding a New Relationship with Your Low Back

I often find that as individuals begin to feel better after a session, they can't wait to begin doing all those things that were put on hold while they were suffering. They find it challenging to allow for the body's healing process and not try to expect too much too soon.

I received a call from a woman who had been in bed for months with a debilitating sciatic pain. After a couple of sessions working together, she began to feel much better. Months of inactivity had caused her muscles to weaken. Concerned about that, I encouraged her to walk for short periods at a time, and to lie down and repeat the pelvic breathing exercises whenever she felt any tension, contraction, or discomfort. After her lower back relaxed, she could get up again and walk for short periods. Interspersing periods of rest and release with walking, the muscles would regain strength, and she would be able to sustain weight bearing for longer periods. Increased activity would be incorporated at a pace that could encourage healing, flexibility, and strength.

She was so excited to be feeling better after months of pain and inactivity that she couldn't contain her desire to be moving. Even though she felt her lower back contract, and tension and discomfort return, she decided that since it was not as bad as before, she would just tough it out. Her impatience short-circuited the healing process, and once again she called from her bed with debilitating pain. We had to start over.

Those individuals who experience a sudden low-back problem may have been enjoying a high level of functioning. Often they are responsible types who not only can take care of themselves but also have stores of energy left over for helping friends. They might think nothing of lifting a sixty-pound box out of the back seat of the car, necessitating a lift and a torque of the spine. They may experience surprise a day or a week later when they reach down to get a carrot out of the bottom drawer of the fridge and find that they can't stand up. Then they may panic. Their schedule is full, time seems limited, and they show up in the office in pain, bent over, wondering how long it will take to fix this, because they have so much to do.

Metaphorically, the low back represents our sense of stability, everything that holds our lives together. A person's low back may "go out" when some stabilizing aspect of life is in flux, such as changing jobs, changing a relationship, or moving from one house to another. Feeling overwhelmed by foundational changes can cause the physical structure to feel overwhelmed, uncertain, and to "go out," so that a person may indeed feel uncertain of what is going to hold him or her up.

While these release positions and exercises help us to recognize that relief from pain is possible, and they assist the body in incorporating newly-found ease and healthier patterns, healing the low back may depend on a bit more than the use of the release positions and movement. There may be unconscious processes at work interrupting the healing or triggering pain responses.[1]

When clients ask how long will it take to heal, my standard reply is, "This will take as long as it takes for you to come into a different kind of relationship with your low back."

Achieving this different relationship may require slowing down and spending some time with yourself, attending to what feels good to your lower back, and noticing which positions bring relief and which movements increase your comfort level.

Anatomy of the Lumbar Spine

The low back is made up of five lumbar vertebrae stacked upon one another, ideally forming a gentle forward (anterior) curve. This part of the spine bears the most weight, so the lumbar vertebrae are the thickest and largest bones of the spine. Gelatinous discs between the vertebral bones act as shock absorbers and allow for movement. The low back is designed mainly for bending forward (flexion) and arching backward (extension), but it allows some side-to-side bending (lateral flexion) and some twisting (rotational) movement. The low back supports the spine and upper torso (Figure 2.1).

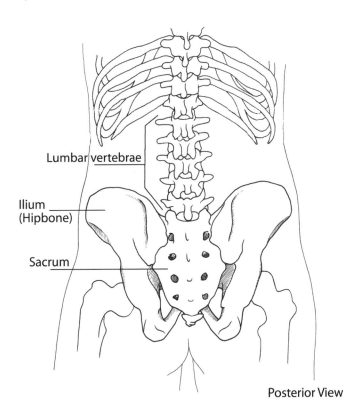

Posterior View

Fig. 2.1. Anatomy of the lumbar spine

LOW BACK GENERAL RELEASE POSITION
WITH ABDOMINAL BREATHING,,,

This is the first exercise I recommend to anyone with low back pain.

Invest twenty minutes resting and breathing in this position. The release position allows your structure to relax any patterns of tension and contraction. Breathing in a slow, even rhythm helps to reestablish a sense of relaxation and well-being.

If possible, try this release a few times throughout the day, especially if back pain or tension is so limiting that you must lie down frequently anyway. If you can only spend ten minutes in this release, let that be okay. Comfortable positioning, focus, breath, and visualization of the exhalation releasing through the low back are key here.

➤ Lie on your back on the floor. Bend your knees and rest your lower legs on a chair or couch. Your heels and lower legs will be resting at knee level or slightly above. Slowly move your knees, one at a time, slightly to the side or closer to your chest, exploring and adjusting until you find just the right position that feels most comfortable for your lower back. Put a pillow under your head if that adds to your comfort (Figure 2.2).

While lying there comfortably, place your hands on your abdomen and inhale slowly and deeply. Your abdomen will rise as breath fills and inflates your lower lungs and then chest. Slowly exhale and the abdomen will fall and soften. Imagine the air leaving gently and slowly through the lower back. Sense the abdomen rising with inhalation and softening at exhalation. Sense the breath moving through the low back during exhalation (Figures 2.3 and 2.4).

Maintain a slow, even pace in both the inhalation and the exhalation. Allow the mouth and lips to be relaxed. Don't blow the air out on exhalation; just let it flow out naturally.

If at any time you experience new discomfort in your low back, move each leg again, slowly, to find your this-very-moment position of comfort.

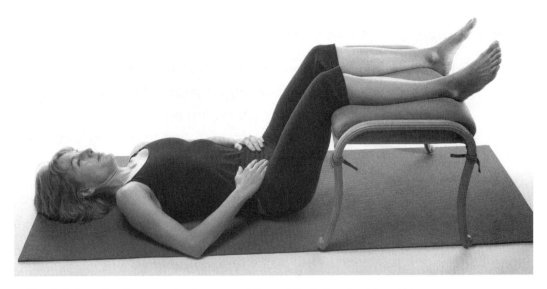

Fig. 2.2. Low back general release position with abdominal breathing

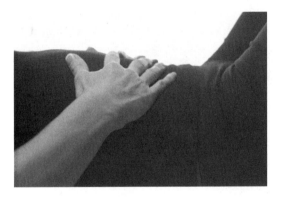

Fig. 2.3. Abdominal breathing: Inhalation

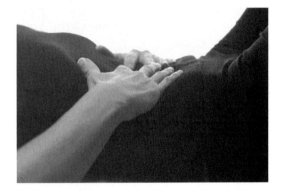

Fig. 2.4. Abdominal breathing: Exhalation

In one instance when this exercise didn't seem to be working, I checked my client's positioning and movement carefully and asked how much time she spent doing this exercise. As it turned out, she was doing the exercise but reading at the same time. I told her that reading interfered with the efficacy of the exercise, but her disappointment turned to delight when I told her she would have to do the exercise for fifteen to twenty minutes without reading and then stay in the position for twenty minutes more to read. Sometimes people with low back pain need a prescription for down time.

※ ※ ※

Anatomy

The thicker lumbar vertebrae are weight-bearing structures for the spine. Weight is transferred from the lumbar vertebrae through the pelvis to our legs for forward movement. When our low back hurts, the tendency is to lock the muscles to feel more supported, and we shorten our potential range of movement.

LOW BACK MOVEMENT: PELVIC CURL WITH BREATHING ,,,

This exercise is good to do after the Abdominal Breathing exercise (above) and/or after the release positions for the 5th Lumbar (below). When we engage in non-weight-bearing movement exercises, we remind the nervous system of the capacity for a relaxed range of movement. We allow the muscles to sense the movement potential without strain from weight and to reorganize toward more functional options.

Stay within your comfort range. If the movement causes pain or strain, make the moves smaller—discover a way to do this that doesn't cause pain.

If you can't find a comfortable way to do it, return to Abdominal Breathing and also try the release positions for the 5th Lumbar. Remember to let your comfort be your guide.

Spend one to ten minutes on this exercise, as long as you are not creating any strain and it feels comfortable for you.

➤ Lie on your back with knees bent and feet on the floor. Line up your knees and feet with the your hips. Begin Abdominal Breathing (see the exercise immediately above)—long, slow inhalations that allow your abdomen to rise—and imagine each exhalation exiting through your low back.

When you have established a relaxed rhythm with your breathing, during an exhalation gently push through your feet, so there is more weight on your soles. Allow the push to transfer through the legs, gently rocking the pelvis and curling the pubic bone up toward the ceiling. As the pubic bone curls up, the low back will flatten toward the floor. If you have trouble with this, try moving your feet a little closer to your buttocks. (If it is still difficult for you, try the Press and Release exercise immediately below.)

As you inhale, slowly release the weight from the feet and allow the abdomen to rise and the pelvis to passively rock back to neutral.

Continue the gentle push-through-feet to curl the pelvis upward during exhalation and to rock back to neutral during inhalation. Allow the abdominal muscles to remain relaxed throughout this exercise, as the breath moves in and out without pressure or forcing (Figures 2.5 and 2.6).

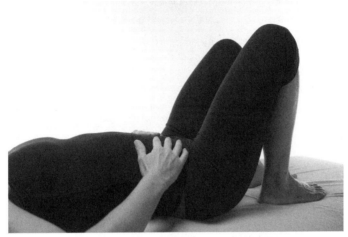

Fig. 2.5. Inhale, weight off feet

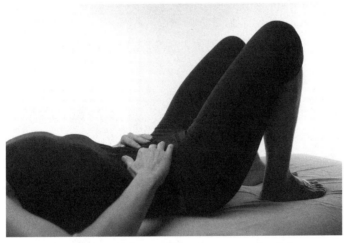

Fig. 2.6. Exhale, push on feet to curl pelvis

If you are having difficulty creating the pelvic curl through pressing into your feet, try this press and release exercise first:

PRESS AND RELEASE[2]
(ASSISTANCE FOR PELVIC CURL EXERCISE ABOVE) ,,

➤ Lie comfortably on your back with knees bent and feet on the floor.

Arch your back slightly and then release it. Gently press your lower back toward the floor and notice how your pubic bone curls up. Then release that movement.

Press your lower back to the floor again, adding a push into your feet, and feel the curling movement supported by the foot pressure. Then see if you can let the pelvic movement come solely from the feet pushing into the floor. (Figures 2.7 and 2.8)

When you've mastered this, add the Abdominal Breathing.

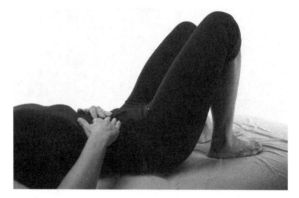

Fig. 2.7. Press the lower back to the floor

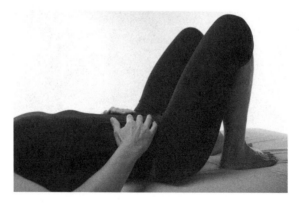

Fig. 2.8. Release the lower back

‰ ‰ ‰

5th Lumbar

Anatomy

The largest and lowest lumbar vertebra is the 5th. It rests on the sacrum (the triangle-shaped bone at the bottom of the spine). This junction is often the seat of low-back pain and the uneasy sense that "the back has gone out." In all cases of low-back pain, spasm, fibromyalgia, and particularly when you can't stand upright, release the 5th lumbar (Figure 2.9).

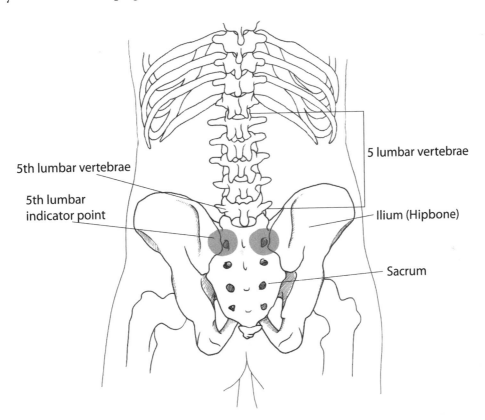

Fig. 2.9. 5th lumbar indicator points

Release Positions for the 5th Lumbar

These two release positions can be repeated at various times throughout the day. Use the one that brings the most relief. As your back begins to relax, and strain and pain are reduced, combine with the Abdominal Breathing, the Pelvic Curl with Breathing exercise (above), and the Supporting the Natural Spinal Curves While You Sleep exercise (Chapter 11) for ongoing maintenance.

➤ Determine which side is tender or painful by checking the indicator points:

- Place your hands on your hips with your thumbs facing toward the spine.

- Walk your thumbs along the top of each hip bone (posterior ilium) as they curve down toward the sacrum.

- Feel for a slight protrusion on the hip bone, called the PSIS, the posterior superior iliac spine (Figure 2.9).

- The indicator point for the 5th lumbar is just inside the posterior edge of this slight protrusion (Figure 2.9). Press out (laterally) on the inside (medial) edge of each bony bump (PSIS). One or both sides can be sore or tender, indicating that the 5th lumbar needs to be released (Figure 2.10).

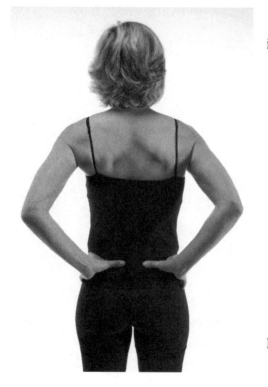

Address whichever side is most sore first. This is called your affected side.

Fig. 2.10. Find the 5th lumbar indicator points

DROPPED LEG ,,,

This release position is usually the most effective for low-back pain, so try it first.

➤ Lie on your abdomen (prone) on the bed with the affected side near the edge. Move your lower body to the edge and your upper body diagonally away, so that you can drop your leg off the side. Your bent knee is pointing to the floor and your foot rests lightly on the floor (Figure 2.11).

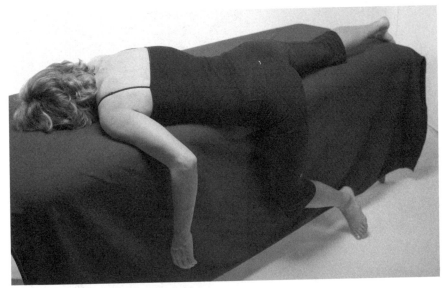

Fig. 2.11. 5th lumbar release position: Dropped Leg

You want to give into gravity, feeling as much of a natural drop from the hip as is possible and comfortable. Do not try to support your weight from your low back, groin area, or dropped leg. If you find that you are holding or if it is difficult for you to relax in this position, you may add some support by placing a chair or cushion under the knee.

Fine-tune the position for maximum comfort. Allow your entire body to relax into this position for a few minutes.

Important: To come out of this release position, slide your other leg off the bed as well, so that you stand up by slowly putting weight onto both feet on the floor. The slide-off approach allows your back to maintain the release and prevents reestablishing the strain pattern. (If you try to lift your dropped leg back onto the bed, you may undo the release and reestablish the tension pattern.) Remember to move into and come out of these positions slowly in order to fine-tune the position and preserve the release (Figures 2.12 to 2.17).

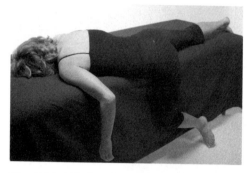

Fig. 2.12. 5th lumbar release position

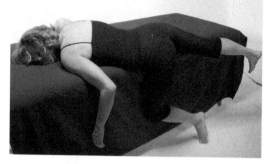

Fig. 2.13. Slide other leg off table

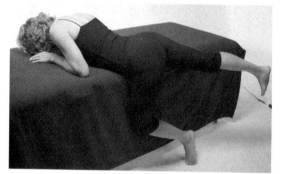

Fig. 2.14. Bring arms up to chest

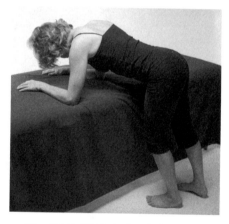

Fig. 2.15. Weight both feet and begin to push up with arms

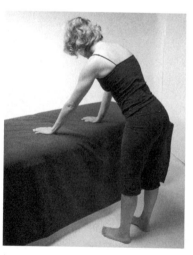
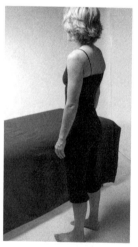

Figs. 2.16 and 2.17. Push up to standing

ALTERNATE RELEASE POSITION FOR 5TH LUMBAR,,

If the Dropped Leg position wasn't comfortable or didn't create release, try this alternative position.

➤ Lie on your abdomen on your bed. Cross the ankle of your *un*affected side (did not have a tender point) over the ankle of the affected side. For support, place a pillow under the hip and thigh of the unaffected side (Figure 2.18).

Maintain this position with the body completely relaxed for a minute or two.

Roll out of the position slowly so as to maintain the release.

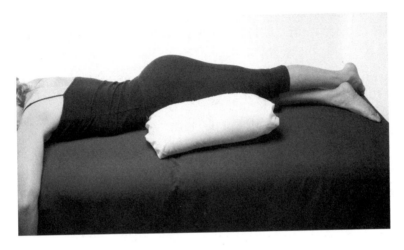

Fig. 2.18. Alternate 5th lumbar release position

⅝ ⅝ ⅝

Isometric/Isotonic Exercises and Stretches for the Lumbar Spine

Isometric and isotonic movement against resistance leads the nervous system to reestablish normal movement function and empowers us to move through restrictive patterning.

These next three exercises interrupt holding patterns that prevent relaxed movement between the lower back, hips, and legs.

These exercises require lying on your side, so find a comfortable (but not squishy) flat surface where you can lie down, stretch out, and move a bit. A comfortable rug on the floor, a yoga mat, or even a bed that is not too soft will work. Use a pillow to support your head and take stress off your neck.

Stay within your range of comfort while doing these exercises. To get the maximum benefit, you must be completely comfortable and pain-free as you do them. If you can't do these movements without pain, don't do them.

ISOMETRIC EXERCISE: UNLOCKING THE LOWER BACK

Some folks have low-back pain because they tend to lock the lower back and not allow hip movement to translate through the low back. The point of this exercise is to open up movement by encouraging a posterior curl in the low back.

➤ Lie on your side. Bend and grasp your knees with both hands. On exhalation, slowly push your knees against your grasp. Feel the movement extending through your hips and pushing the lower back out away from the knees. It's important to feel the movement of pushing into your knees translate through the pelvis, curling your pubic bone forward and creating a rounding movement of the low back (Figure 2.19).

Slowly release your grasp and allow your legs to straighten, completing the movement they were trying to make.

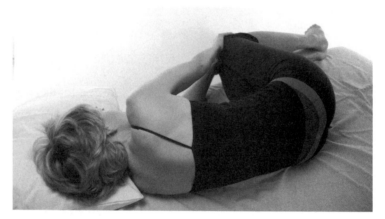

Fig. 2.19. Knee push for posterior curl of the low back

POSITION AND ISOTONIC: SIDE-BENDING MOVEMENT (LATERAL FLEXION) IN LOWER BACK ,,

➤ Lie on your side with your knees bent at a 90-degree angle, to be even with your hips. With your knees remaining in place, slowly raise your feet and ankles up toward the ceiling, and then lower them. Notice the comfort level of your lower back as you do this movement. If comfortable, repeat a few times (Figure 2.20).

Does your lower back feel better with the feet and ankles raised? If so, this is your "comfortable position." Support the feet and ankles on a cushion in the comfortable position, and rest like that for a couple of minutes (Figure 2.21).

Initiate an isotonic movement: Gently push your feet and ankles down through the cushion (Figure 2.22). Remove the cushion and repeat the ankle-lift movement (Figure 2.20). Check for comfort and ease.

Repeat this position and isotonic on the other side. Notice if it is easier on one side than the other. If so, always do the exercise on the easier side first, which helps to release and balance it with the other side.

Another variation of this is to hold your ankles and give yourself resistance as you attempt to push the feet down for seven to ten seconds. As with any isometric, release and allow the feet to complete the attempted movement. You can also vary the stretch by bending the knees at different angles (Figures 2.23 and 2.24).

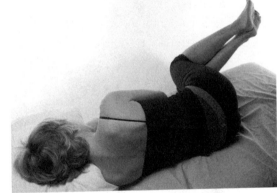

Fig. 2.20. Lift feet for side flexion of low back (low-back side bend)

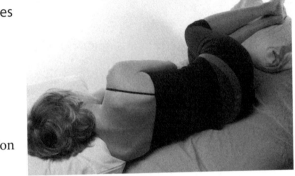

Fig. 2.21. Lateral flexion (side bend) release position for low back

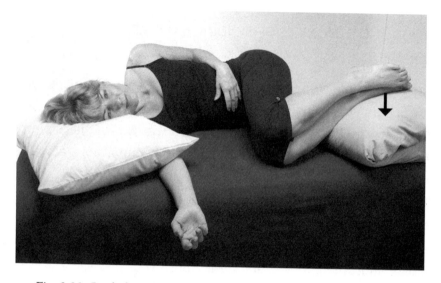

Fig. 2.22. Push feet through pillow toward floor for ten seconds

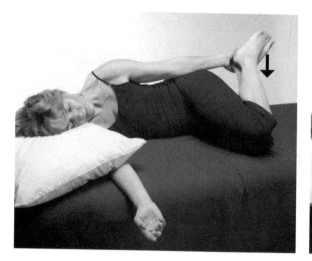
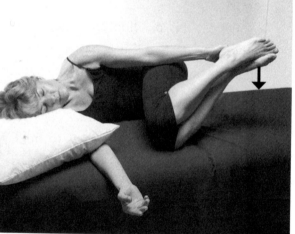

Figs. 2.23 and 2.24. Variation isometric with different angles of knee bend

RELAXED ROTATIONAL STRETCH FOR LOW-BACK FLEXIBILITY,,,,,,,,,,,,,,,,,,,,,,,,,

➤ Lying on your side, straighten the bottom leg and bend the top leg, so that the top knee drops slightly in front of the bottom leg.

Rest your top arm on the side of your torso, and allow that shoulder and arm to slowly drop back toward the floor into a comfortable stretch (Figure 2.25).

Rest and relax your whole body in this position. Remember to continue breathing fully. Allow your head to gently turn toward the top shoulder. Does this allow your shoulder to relax down even more (Figure 2.26)?

You can also extend your arm up above your head for another stretch. Repeat on your other side.

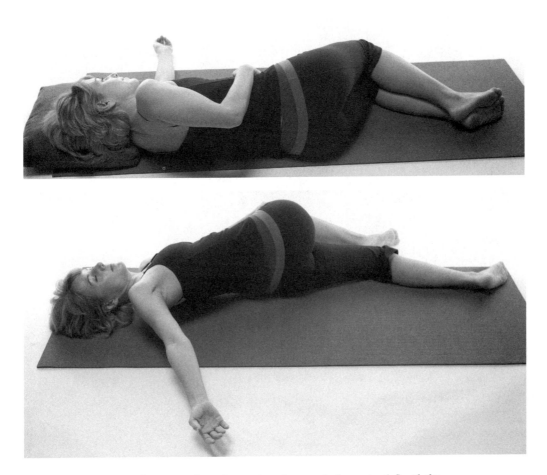

Figs. 2.25 and 2.26. Relaxed rotational stretch for spinal flexibility

❧ ❧ ❧

CHAPTER 3

Pelvis: Sacrum, Hips, Sacroiliac Joint, and Tailbone

Marianne's Story: Pelvic Thyroid Syndrome

While I was giving a lecture-demonstration in Australia, a woman volunteered to experience a demonstration of Ortho-Bionomy. Marianne, a massage therapist, was looking for new skills to add to her practice. When I asked her what she would like me to address in the session, she explained that she had been experiencing some low-back problems recently and that her voice had become raspy. Even though she no longer had a cold, her voice had not returned to normal. She suspected a thyroid problem, but medical tests showed that her thyroid was within normal ranges. She said she wanted her normal voice back.

I explained that sometimes when the pelvis and low back become unbalanced, the reflexes to the organs and glands get thrown off.[1] When I checked and found a discrepancy in Marianne's leg lengths, she told me about an injury and resultant surgery that left one leg shorter. She had a lift for her shoe but recently hadn't been wearing it.

Through the positioning releases for her low back, particularly the 5th lumbar release and hip (ilium) releases, we were able to gain more range of movement and flexibility in her lower back. Then we worked with the upper back using positioning to release tender points alongside her spine. Next we used positioning releases for her shoulders and clavicle. Finally, after twenty minutes, we ended by releasing the neck and checking the movement preference for her hyoid bone at her throat and releasing the tension there.

Marianne stood up and began to describe how much better she was feeling in her lower back, and then she suddenly noticed, "I have my voice back. This is my normal voice." I think everyone there was surprised that her voice had changed so quickly.

Through my studies I have learned that we can't always expect such immediate results as Marianne's. Often problems in the body are the result of years of postural misalignments and compensations, and so the process of reeducation and realignment can take some time.

The reflexes that save us from a fall as we trip over a curb are part of our proprioceptive sense. This proprioceptive sense is a network of nerve responses that provide information about the position of the body and assist in coordinating and regulating all of our movement responses. This network of self-balancing reflexes has a memory of what works best for functionality. We can thank these proprioceptive reflexes when we walk up stairs and don't have to think about how high to lift our foot with each step.

Sometimes, however, after that fall off the curb, our reflexes don't quite reset back to normal. Instead we develop holding or compensation patterns that alter the usual way our body moves. Our proprioceptive sense now incorporates the compensation pattern and remembers it. But the original memory of functionality lies under the compensation pattern and can be accessed and reset through positioning and gentle compression. The timing of how rapidly this reset can happen depends on how long we have been using the compensation pattern and thereby normalizing it, and on the health and responsiveness of our reflexes.

Marianne's story illustrates that the pelvis and low back are the foundation for structural and functional integrity. The entire structural memory is addressed by releasing the various tension and holding patterns with positioning. Her reflexive balance returned spontaneously once the body remembered its foundational and functional integrity.

Anatomy: Sacrum, Hips, Sacroiliac Joint, Quadratus Lumborum, and Tailbone

The pelvis is a bowl formed by the sacrum (the triangle-shaped bone at the bottom of our spine) and flanked on each side by a disc-shaped hip bone (ilium). The tailbone (coccyx) attaches to the end of the sacrum and normally curves under a bit (Figure 3.1). On each side of the sacrum is a joint formed where the sacrum and ilium meet. Strong ligaments bind this sacroiliac joint together but allow a slight rocking movement between the sacrum and the two hip bones (Figure 3.2). Each hip bone (ilium) has a fused connection with the sit bone (ischium) on the same side, which in turn has a fused connection with the pubic bone. These structures create the pelvic bowl (Figure 3.1).

Each hip bone also forms the socket structure for the ball or head of the thigh bone (femur). The pelvic bones, along with the ligaments and muscles that attach to them, form a support for our internal organs, stability for sitting, and flexibility for walking.

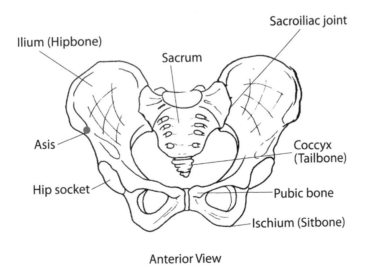

Anterior View

Fig. 3.1. Female pelvis (front/anterior view). Extract from *Anatomy of Movement,* courtesy of Blandine Calais Germain and Désiris Publishing, France.

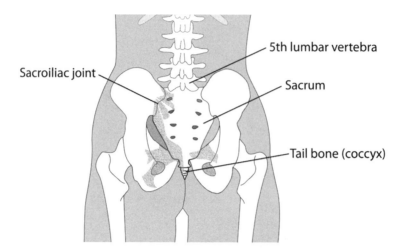

Fig. 3.2. Posterior Pelvis with Sacral Ligaments

Sacrum

The sacrum serves as a transition place. The weight of the spine rests on the sacrum and is transferred diagonally through the sacrum to the hip sockets and down the legs to the feet. When we walk, the spring from each step alternately moves up each leg and through the hip socket to the sacroiliac joint, transferring the movement up the spine and allowing the sacrum to gently rock between the hip bones.

Injury or repeated use patterns sometimes cause the sacroiliac joint to become locked or tight, limiting the movement of the sacrum or the hips. If the sciatic nerve becomes irritated from this imbalance, it can result in pain in the hip that may radiate down the leg, commonly known as sciatica (see Chapter 17).

The word "sacrum" means "sacred." So in working with the sacrum, treat yourself gently and with respect.

The sacrum forms a type of shield, and the bowl of the pelvis creates a protective structure for the organs of physical creation. The uterus sits directly in front of the sacrum, so tension around the sacrum can translate to tension around the uterus.

This exercise to release the sacrum and the ones for the sacroiliac joint (presented below) can also help with menstrual pain. Sometimes pressure on the sacrum helps with labor during childbirth.

Anatomy of the Sacrum

The sacrum is made up of five vertebral bones fused into the shape of a triangle that has a slight posterior curve. Its top vertebral bone, known as S1, forms a joint with the 5th lumbar vertebra, L5; the lowest vertebral bone, S5, forms a joint with the tailbone (coccyx). See Figure 3.3.

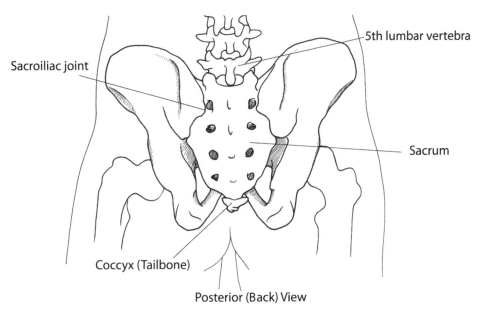

Fig. 3.3. Sacrum

GENERAL RELEASE FOR THE SACRUM ///

Use sacrum release in combination with hip bone and 5th lumbar releases and sacroiliac exercises. Also see Chapter 17 for more sciatica exercises.

➤ Lying on your back, place a soft, hollow, rubber ball (about the size of a large grapefruit) under your sacrum. Slowly roll around on the ball, exploring for positions that give comfortable pressure into the sacrum. Remember that comfort is your guide, so find the angles of no pain (Figure 3.4).

Allow yourself three to five minutes for this exercise.

If you are not comfortable doing this exercise, skip it. Something else might need to be addressed first.

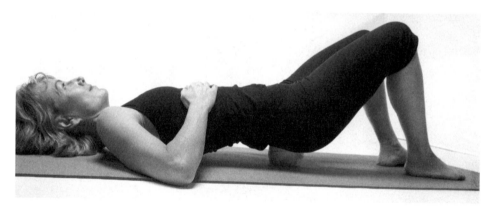

Fig. 3.4. Sacrum ball

⁂

Hips

I once worked with an elderly gentleman of the ripe old age of ninety-two. He said that he was doing fine, except it always felt like he was walking with one foot up on a curb. Along with protective muscle spasms, his hip bone (ilium) was rotated such that he had a one-inch leg length discrepancy.

As we saw with the case of Marianne, a hip rotation can reflexively upset a person's balance on many levels—even affecting the endocrine system. Injury or repeated use patterns can cause the sacroiliac joint to get stuck, with compensation patterns resulting in discomfort in the lower back, the knees, or even in the shoulders. If the sciatic nerve becomes irritated from this imbalance, it can result in pain in the hip that may radiate down the leg, commonly known as sciatica. (For more information on sciatica, see Chapter 17.)

Pelvic balance is vital, and much of it depends on balanced hips. It all may seem complex, but if we check the reflex (indicator) points for tenderness then address each of the areas in turn, we begin to open up movement options and opportunities for self-correction.

If you begin to get relief from these positional releases and exercises but the pain returns, it could be that the problem is coming from a repetitive pattern of use at work or in the way you walk or sit. It is important to remember that factors contributing to a pelvis or hip problem can be found in repeated use patterns that have also affected the lumbar vertebrae above, or the feet, knees, and legs below. You may need to address those areas as well.

For example, a contractor came for relief of nagging lower-back pain. He would do the release positions and feel better for a couple of days after the session, but the pain would return. I reasoned that he was using his body at work in a way that was reestablishing the pain pattern. We finally determined that the tool belt he wore around his waist pulled his hips forward. He turned his tool belt around and wore it on the back for half the day. By adapting a new pattern of use, his muscles strengthened more evenly and worked in a more functionally balanced way. This simple solution allowed him to stay balanced and work without pain.

Anatomy of the Hip Bone (Ilium)

The ilium is better known as the hip bone. These are the bones we contact when we put our hands on our hips at the sides of the pelvis (Figure 3.5). Each hip bone has a fused connection with the sit bone (ischium) at the bottom. The sit bone, in turn, has a fused connection through a narrow bone (ramus) along the inside of the leg with the pubic bone in front. Each hip bone provides the structure for the socket that houses the ball of the femur at the top of the leg.

As we walk, the hip bones rock forward and back slightly. A slip on the stair or off a curb can cause an ilium to lose its mobility. Depending on which muscles and ligaments tighten to catch us, the ilium can be stuck in either a slight forward (anterior) or backward (posterior) rotation, causing an uneven leg length.

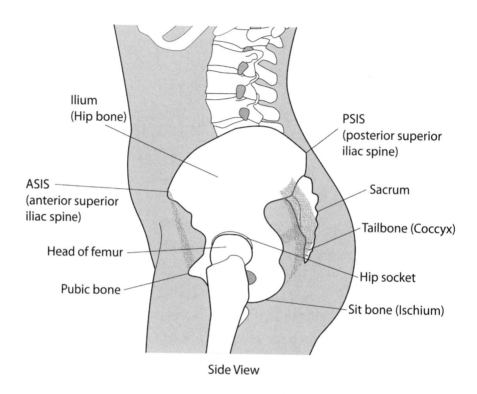

Side View

Fig. 3.5. Hip bone (side view of ilium)

Assessing Rotation of the Hip Bone (Ilium)

When a hip bone rotates back (posteriorly) and gets stuck in a posterior rotation, the leg appears shorter on that side. When a hip bone rotates forward (anteriorly) and gets stuck in an anterior rotation, that leg will seem longer (Figures 3.6 and 3.7).

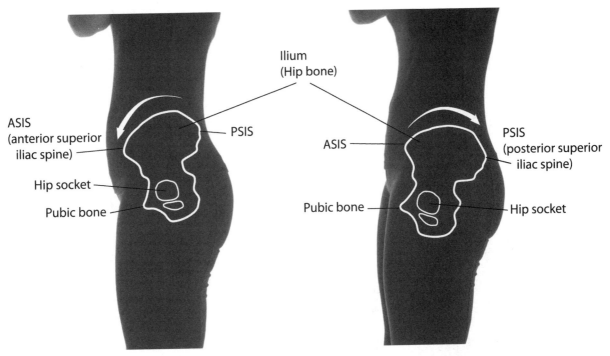

Fig. 3.6. Anterior rotation of hip bone   Fig. 3.7. Posterior rotation of hip bone

If you have an uneven leg length and are unsure whether it's due to an anterior rotation causing a long leg or a posterior rotation causing a short leg, you may do the releases for both and see which one feels better.

You may also check for tenderness at the reflex point to determine the side that is affected and, therefore, the side that needs to be addressed. This point for a rotated ilium is located on both sides on the upper part of the buttock, about an inch to an inch-and-a-half diagonally down from the PSIS (posterior superior iliac spine). See Figures 3.8 and 3.9.

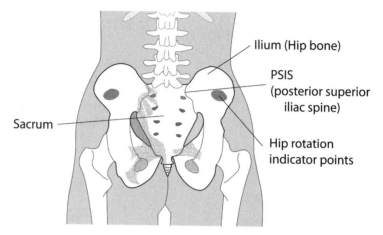

Fig. 3.8. Hip (ilium) rotation indicator points

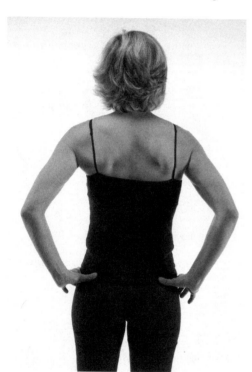

Fig. 3.9. Find hip rotation indicator points

Another way to assess is to feel for restriction of movement at the hip bones on the front of the body.

➤ Lie on your back and place one hand on the front of each hip bone at the anterior superior iliac spine, also known as the ASIS (Figure 3.10). Using both of your hands, feel if the two sides are even. Push back slightly on one hip and then the other to see if one side seems resistant to movement or has more capacity to move backwards or to rebound from your push. If one side feels more anterior (higher toward the ceiling) than the other and doesn't seem to have much give when you push, then treat this as an anterior rotation, especially if this leg seems longer. The side that is lower and pushes back easily could be a posterior rotation (Figure 3.11).

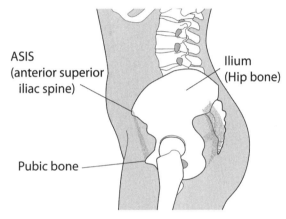

Fig. 3.10. ASIS of hip

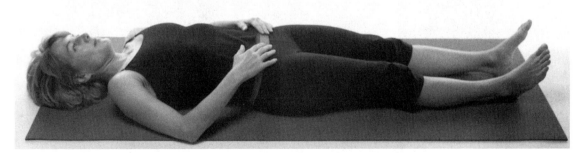

Fig. 3.11. Sensing height and movement potential at the ASIS
(front hip bones)

RELEASE POSITION FOR A POSTERIOR ROTATION OF THE HIP (SHORTER LEG): FROG POSITION

Posterior rotations tend to be most common and usually result in a shorter leg on the same side. Check for tenderness at the indicator point as well.

Remember these release positions slightly exaggerate the direction in which the hip is stuck. So if you have a short leg you will "shorten" it further by bending the knee into the "frog" position. This will rotate the hip of the short leg more posterior. If you have a long leg you will bring the ilium (hip bone) slightly more anterior with the release position. Try this release for cases of sciatica along with the release for the 5th lumbar.

➤ Lie on your abdomen and slowly bend your knee, bringing it out to the side of your body. This will rotate the hip a bit more posterior. We refer to this as the Frog position (Figure 3.12).

Turn your head to the same side as the knee is pointing. A pillow may be placed under the raised hip for support.

Allow the entire body to relax in this position for a few minutes. Be sure to be comfortable. If you aren't, don't continue in the position.

Remember to come out of this position very slowly so as not to reestablish the old holding pattern.

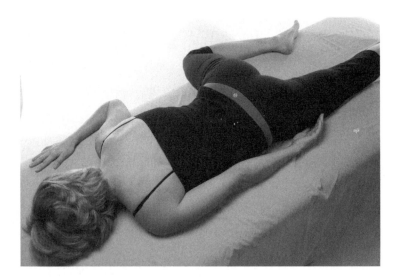

Fig. 3.12. Frog position to release posterior hip rotation

※ ※ ※

RELEASE POSITION FOR AN ANTERIOR ROTATION
OF THE HIP (LONGER LEG) ,,,

With an anterior rotation of the hip, the leg is seen as longer, or the front bony curve of that hip (ASIS) may feel higher (more anterior) when you are lying on your back.

For sciatica, try this position if the Frog position doesn't help. Combine with the low back releases and particularly the 5th lumbar release positions.

➤ Stand at the corner at the end of a bed and rest your upper thigh and knee on the bed. Place your hands on the bed and support your upper body on your fully extended arms. Allow the front of the hip bone (ASIS) to drop slightly toward the bed. This will rotate the hip a bit more anterior. You may need to bend your standing knee a little. Maintain this position, if comfortable for the hip, for ten to thirty seconds (Figure 3.13).

You may also release the leg by lying on the bed on your abdomen and placing a pillow under your thigh for support as the hip is rotated slightly more anterior (Figure 3.14).

Remember to come out of the position slowly.

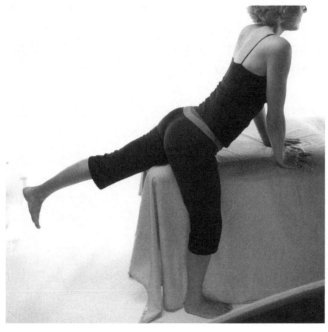

Fig. 3.13. Release position for longer leg (anterior hip rotation)

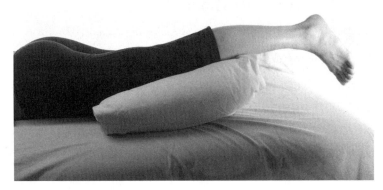

Fig. 3.14. Exaggerate the forward position of the anterior hip,
using a pillow for support

※ ※ ※

Sacroiliac Joint

The sacrum forms a joint with each hip bone called the sacroiliac joint (Figure 3.15). Tension or imbalance at this joint can cause sciatic pain as well as menstrual pain, or may contribute to a hormonal disorder. Do the release positions for the hip, the low back (particularly the 5th lumbar), and the sacrum. Once the joint is open you can maintain its flexibility by doing the following movement exercises daily. Keeping this joint balanced and flexible is essential to balanced posture and good endocrine health.[2]

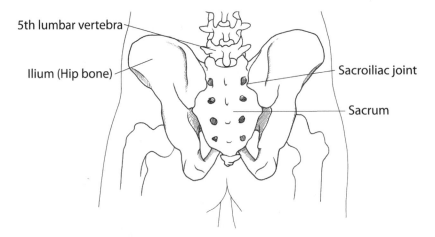

Fig. 3.15. Sacroiliac joint (meeting of hip with sacrum)

Movement Exercises to Maintain Flexibility in the Sacroiliac Joint

Walking is one of the most useful activities for pain in the sacrum and sacroiliac region. Instead of going to bed to rest when you feel discomfort or tension in this area, take a short walk. Walking can be a very effective way to remind the body of its natural capacity to return balance to this area. More information on walking can be found in the Chapter 9.

The following exercises also help to bring balance and maintain flexibility in the sacroiliac joint. As you do these movements, put your attention on your sacroiliac joints. All these exercises can be used to relieve menstrual cramps, especially if done regularly.

TEENAGE TELEPHONE TALK ⁄⁄⁄

➤ Lying on your abdomen (prone), bend your knees so your feet are up in the air. Slowly draw circles in the air with your feet, noting where in the circle there is more ease and comfort. You may pause and rest in any comfortable positions for a few moments.

This exercise is named Teenage Telephone Talk because it captures the mood of a relaxed teen, unconsciously self-balancing the pelvis while chatting on the phone (Figure 3.16).

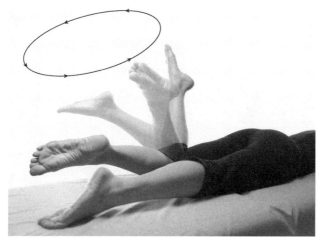

Fig. 3.16. Teenage Telephone Talk: Foot Circles

SCISSORS ///

➤ Lying on your abdomen, bend your knees and let the feet swing out to the sides and then toward each other, crossing the midline like scissors (Figures 3.17 to 3.19).

Keep your movements slow and easy—this is not an aerobic workout.

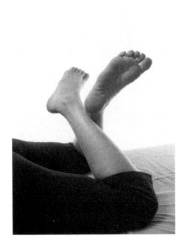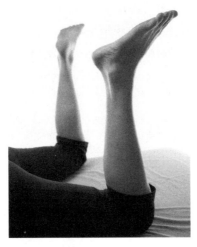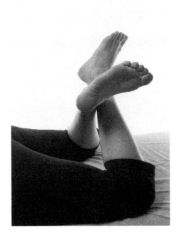

Figs. 3.17 to 3.19. Scissors

FOOT AND LEG RUB ⁄⁄

This exercise increases flexibility in the sacroiliac joint.

➤ Lie on your abdomen with your knees bent and your feet in the air.

Rub your feet against each other, touching all the surfaces together. Remember to include the tops and sides of the feet. Notice if one foot is more active in the rubbing movement than the other, and balance the movement action between the feet.

Then rub down the inside of each leg with the opposing foot (Figures 3.20 to 3.23).

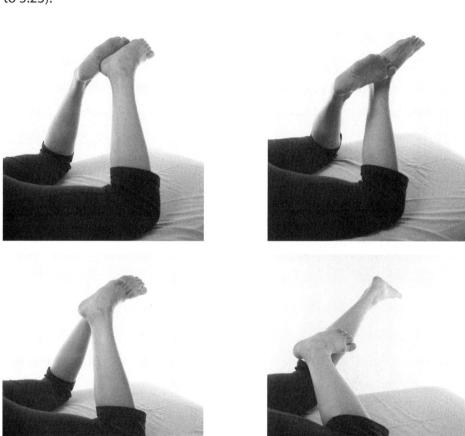

Figs. 3.20 to 3.23. Foot and Leg Rub for sacroiliac flexibility

⁊ ⁊ ⁊

Quadratus Lumborum: Connecting the Low Back and the Pelvis

Often pain or tension in the low back is caused by a rotational injury, as in the case of the client who lifted and twisted while moving a sixty-pound box out of the back seat of her car. For this, you may need a position that allows you to shorten the tight and contracted muscle between the hip and the lower back.

Anatomy of the Quadratus Lumborum

The quadratus lumborum (QL) is a deep-lying back muscle. It is addressed here because of its relationship to the hip. The QL extends from the crest of the hip bone to the 12th rib and attaches to each lumbar vertebra (Figure 3.24). The QL muscle side-bends (laterally flexes) the trunk of the body. If the low back is locked up, this muscle can raise or "hike up" the hip. If the pelvis is not moving properly this muscle can pull the lumbar spine and rib cage into a side-bend curve as can happen in scoliosis. So be sure to address this area after you get the hip bones and low back released and when needed in cases of scoliosis.

You can assess for tightness in this area by placing your hands on your hips with thumbs forward and fingers of each hand fanning the space between the top of your hip and your lumbar vertebrae (Figures 3.25 and 3.26).

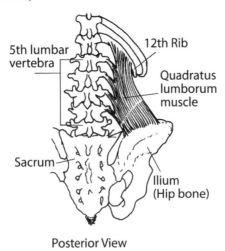

5th lumbar vertebra

12th Rib

Quadratus lumborum muscle

Sacrum

Ilium (Hip bone)

Posterior View

Fig. 3.24. Quadratus Lumborum (QL) muscle

Courtesy of *Illustrated Essentials of Musculoskeletal Anatomy,* 4th Edition by Sieg and Adams (Gainesville, FL: Megabooks, Inc., 1992), www.muscleanatomybook.com.

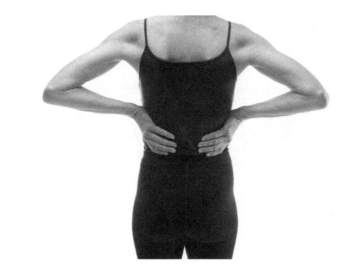

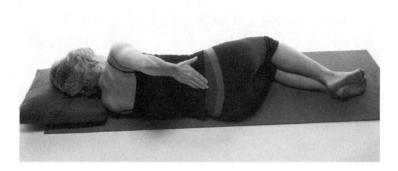

Figs. 3.25 and 3.26. Sensing for tension in the area
of the quadratus lumborum

RELEASING THE QUADRATUS LUMBORUM: THE LAZY DOG ,,,,,,,,,,,,,,,,,,,,,,,,,,,,,,

Use this release position for tension in the low back between the ribs and
hips.

➤ Lie on your side on the floor with your knees bent. Be sure that your
hips, shoulders, and head are in a straight line. Support your head with a pillow (Figure 3.27).

Place a chair behind you, just at the level of your thighs, with the seat of
the chair facing the back of your thighs. With your elbow resting on your side
at your waist, slowly roll back and place your calf on the chair behind you. This

creates a slight rotation in your low back that relaxes the triangular-shaped area between your low back and your hip (the quadratus lumborum muscle).

Check with your hand to sense the tissue softening in this area.

Allow your elbow to slide back toward the floor.

In this release position it is important that your upper buttock falls back toward the floor but does not actually rest completely on the floor. You want to allow the lower area of your back to relax and feel suspended while the lower leg is supported on the chair. It is also important that your hips, shoulders, and head are aligned with the edge of the chair. In other words, don't curl the top of your body forward (Figure 3.28).

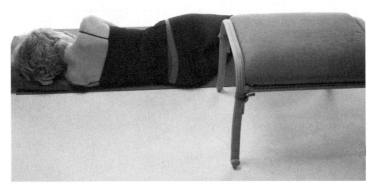

Fig. 3.27. Set-up for Lazy Dog release

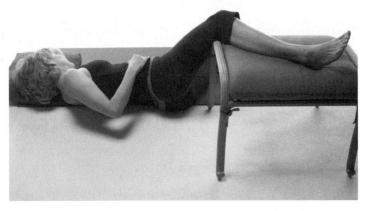

Fig. 3.28. Lazy Dog release position for QL

MOVEMENT EXERCISE TO MAINTAIN FLEXIBILITY
IN THE QUADRATUS LUMBORUM

After you have released the quadratus lumborum area of the low back, you can maintain the flexibility and mobility in this area with this simple movement exercise.

➤ Begin in the same position as above, lying on your side on the floor with your knees bent. Your hips, shoulders, and head are in a straight line, and your head is supported on a pillow. Your elbow is resting on your side. Open and close the top leg by raising and lowering the knee. The foot stays on the floor.

As you raise the knee, allow the hip to open and the upper body to fall slightly back toward the floor. As the knee closes, the hip and spine return to the original aligned position. It is important for the upper body to follow the movement of the hip. In other words, do not initiate movement from the upper body (Figures 3.29 to 3.32).

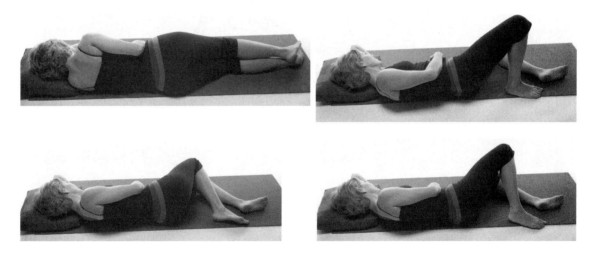

Figs. 3.29 to 3.32. Open and close the upper leg
to release the low back in the area of the quadratus lumborum

✥ ✥ ✥

Tailbone

Tension or tenderness at the tailbone (coccyx) can cause discomfort when we sit and can sometimes be a contributing factor in sciatic pain. Be sure to do the releases for the sacrum, hips, and 5th lumbar as well as this subtle technique to release pain at the tailbone.

The tailbone is the very end of the spine, at the bottom of the triangle-shaped sacrum. The curl of the coccyx consists of even smaller, fused vertebrae and is held in place by ligaments connecting it to the sacrum (Figure 3.33).

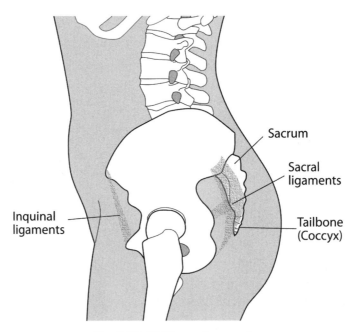

Fig. 3.33. Tailbone (coccyx)

TAILBONE RELEASE///

In this release you will be contacting a reflex point near the left wrist as well as any area of tension around the tailbone.

➤ First find the reflex point on the thumb side of your left forearm, about one or two inches above the wrist. Palpate between the bones of the forearm, applying pressure to the back of the radius (the bone on the thumb side of the arm) until you find a sore and/or tender point (Figure 3.34).

Then, standing, reach around with your left hand and gently contact the tailbone with your middle finger. Softly touch the tissue on both sides of the tailbone and check for tenderness on the bone itself. Note any tension or tightness in the area and monitor it with your left middle finger. Then, reach your right hand around your back and contact the forearm point of your left arm with your right middle finger (Figure 3.35).

Now, very lightly press on the wrist point and lighten your contact with the monitoring finger on your tailbone, wait a few seconds, then let the pressure on the wrist relax as you lightly press on the tailbone point. Very slowly, alternate pressure on the two points until all tenderness and tension release (Figure 3.36).

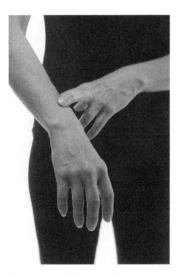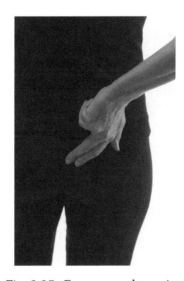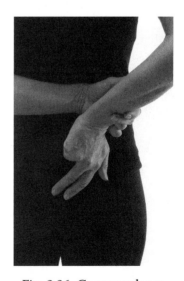

Fig. 3.34. Wrist reflex point   Fig. 3.35. Coccyx tender point   Fig. 3.36. Coccyx release

⁊ ⁊ ⁊

CHAPTER 4

Alignment of Hips, Legs, Knees, and Feet

Various phrases comment on our relationship with this area of the body: The hips, legs, and feet are responsible for our "stance in the world," "how we move forward in life," how we "walk our talk," whether we "stand on our own two feet," or "shoot straight from the hip." Each points to the importance of alignment. A car won't get you very far if you mount the front tires at a forty-five-degree angle instead of aligned forward. Just like tires, the hips, legs, ankles, and feet need to be aligned so they function optimally and don't wear out prematurely.

Check the Alignment of Your Feet

➤ Stand and look down at the position of your feet. Are the toes pointed straight ahead or do your feet angle slightly out to the sides like misaligned tires? If you notice that they turn out, it is important to realize that forcing your feet to go forward won't change the pattern. Doing that would only cause further tensions throughout all the relationships between the feet and hips (Figures 4.1 and 4.2).

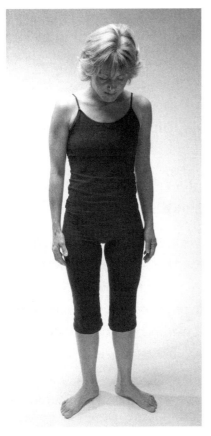

Fig. 4.1. Angled feet

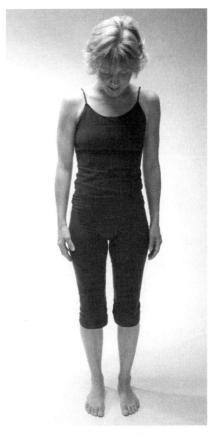

Fig. 4.2. Parallel feet

Exaggerating and Reeducating the Pattern with Simple Movements

➤ In Ortho-Bionomy, we recommend that you walk for one minute in an exaggeration of the turned-out pattern; in other words, walk with your feet turned out even further (like a penguin). This exaggeration helps the body to recognize the pattern and relax it.

Next, consciously walk with your feet parallel for another minute. This offers another option to your proprioceptive senses.

Now forget about it. Forgetting about it keeps you from trying to hold onto a correction. The body can then integrate the new option at a functional pace.

Repeat this exercise sequence frequently throughout the day to begin to release the restrictive patterning and drop pebbles of possibility into the proprioceptive nervous system, small reminders to the self-corrective reflexes.

In these simple movement exercises, notice how quickly change can occur just by spending a few seconds affirming your movement preference.

KNEE ROCKING AFTER HIP REPLACEMENT SURGERY

A delightful, courageous woman with a lovely sense of humor came to my office. In her late sixties, she had had replacement surgeries on both hips. After the surgery, she had fallen and her right femur had slipped out of the socket, yet she clearly decided that she was much too fragile for any more surgery. Instead, she elected to walk with a two-inch lift on her shoe. The resulting unevenness of her leg lengths despite the two-inch lift, as well as residual tension from the fall, caused restrictions and holding patterns throughout her body. These tension patterns caused pain and limited her movement capacity.

When I asked what bothered her most, she said she had pain every time she stood up from a sitting position. I suggested that she gently rock her knees side to side a few times before she stood up. This would allow any tension or holding patterns to get accustomed to movement before the area became weight bearing. It also would increase proprioception in her knees, ankles, and hips. By bringing her attention to the area and self-regulating the movement before weight bearing, she prepared the muscles around the joint for weight-bearing movement. The rocking movements she made while still sitting indeed stimulated her proprioception and increased her coordination and cohesion from her hips down through her feet. She was then able to move from sitting to standing without pain.

Additionally, by working with what is functional, she created connections between the body's various neighborhoods and extended functionality, as each area related better with the next.

SIDE-TO-SIDE BALANCE ⫽⫽⫽

➤ Stand with your feet parallel about two to three inches apart. Shift your hips, and therefore your weight on your feet, laterally from one side to the other.

Notice which side feels more comfortable and shift to that side.

Wait there for ten to thirty seconds, move back to center, and recheck for balance side to side (Figures 4.3 and 4.4).

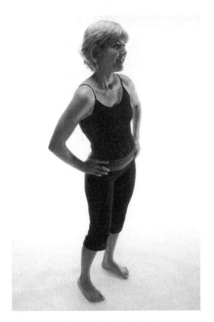
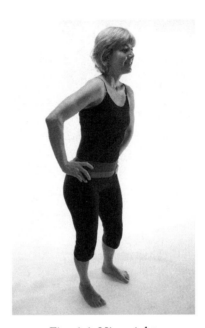

Fig. 4.3. Hips left   Fig. 4.4. Hips right

FORWARD AND BACK BALANCE ⫽⫽⫽⫽⫽⫽⫽⫽⫽⫽⫽⫽⫽⫽⫽⫽⫽⫽⫽⫽⫽⫽⫽⫽⫽⫽⫽⫽⫽⫽⫽⫽⫽⫽⫽⫽⫽

➤ Starting in the same position as above, shift your weight forward and back. Notice if you feel more comfortable with your weight on the front of your feet or toward your heels.

Move to the more comfortable position and hold this position for ten to thirty seconds.

Then shift back to center and recheck for balance front to back (Figures 4.5 and 4.6).

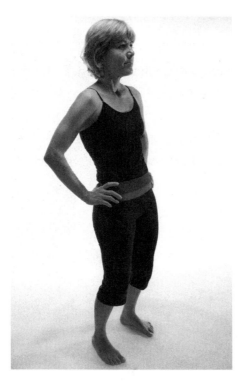

Fig. 4.5. Hips forward

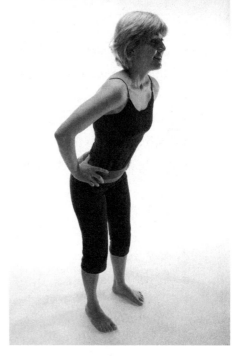

Fig. 4.6. Hips back

ROTATING THE PELVIS

➤ Rotate your pelvis in a circular direction, exploring preferences and noting any discomfort or glitches in movement.

Move in a circle to a position directly opposite any discomfort or glitch—which should be comfortable—and stay in that position ten to thirty seconds.

Then rotate the pelvis again to recheck. If there has been no change in the discomfort, stop the movement directly before the glitch and hold this posture ten to thirty seconds. Then recheck (Figures 4.7 to 4.10).

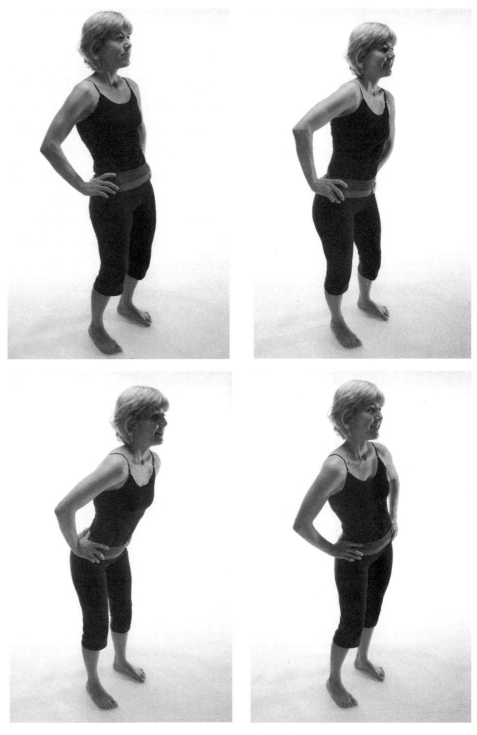

Figs. 4.7 to 4.10. Rotate the pelvis in a circle

Femur

The femur, the tibia, and the fibula are the three bones of the leg. Weight is transferred down the spine through the pelvic hip sockets and into the legs for balance and forward movement. Proper alignment of these bones assists in balanced weight transfer through the legs and functional use of the muscles for walking, standing and movement. This alignment begins at the femur (thigh bone).

The long thigh bone (femur) extends from the hip socket to the knee. The top of the femur is spherical, and with the pelvis it forms a ball-and-socket joint. This provides an extraordinary range of motion while balancing the weight of the torso. At the lower end, the femur joins with the larger lower leg bone, called the tibia, and forms the knee joint (Figure 4.11).

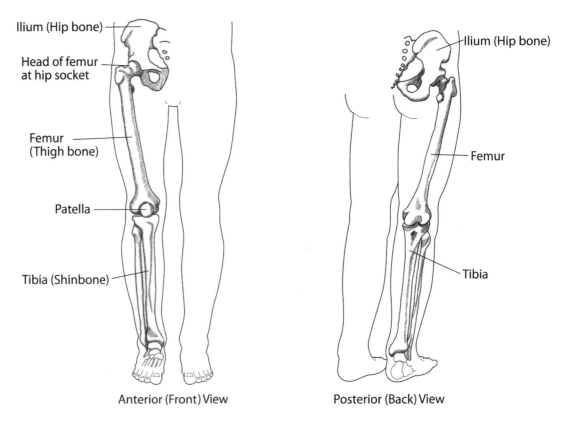

Ilium (Hip bone)

Head of femur at hip socket

Femur (Thigh bone)

Patella

Tibia (Shinbone)

Ilium (Hip bone)

Femur

Tibia

Anterior (Front) View

Posterior (Back) View

Fig. 4.11. Anatomy of the leg

The alignment of hips, knees, ankles, and feet supports the weight-bearing and movement capacity of the lower body and allows the knees to function with ease and stability. The weight of the body is optimally carried through the bones. The weight of the spine is transferred through the sacrum to the hips and hip sockets, then to the femur and tibia, and finally to the talus and bones of the foot.

Awareness Exercise for the Hips and Legs

I was introduced to Gerda Alexander[1], one of my early teachers, when she was advanced in age. Director of a school in Copenhagen, she taught students to heal injuries using her simple principles of self-care. Although I had the privilege of studying with her for only a short time, that experience and training deeply influenced my attitude and approach toward self-care. Each of her exercises led me to a direct experience of the intelligence of the body and increased my internal awareness and understanding of my own functionality.

INITIATING MOVEMENT FROM DIFFERENT PLACES ,,,

This exercise with the knee demonstrated to me that the specific area from which movement is initiated can alter the way the body organizes the movement. Initiating the same directional movement from different places on the same joint can offer the body another option to a painful movement pattern.

Try this movement exercise for yourself and notice how many options you have for making a movement. This exercise can be very subtle, so slow down and place your attention on the area from which you are initiating the movement.

➤ Lie on your back with knees bent and feet resting flat on the floor.

Raise your left knee toward your chest and rub only the *front* of your knee with your hand to increase your sensation in that area. Then return the foot to resting flat on the floor.

Sense the front of your knee where you have just rubbed, and focus your attention on that sensation as you initiate a movement *from the front of the knee* toward the foot. Really get the sense that the front of the knee is leading the movement toward the foot and the rest of the leg is following. Now—still initiating from the front of the knee—slowly bring the knee back away from the foot to its original position (Figures 4.12 and 4.13).

Next, rub the *outside* (lateral area) of the left knee to increase the sensation. Place your attention on this outside area of the left knee and initiate from there to move the knee toward the foot (same direction as before, just the initiation point changes). Sense the outside of the left knee leading the movement forward toward the foot. Notice if and in what way the movement feels different from the previous time. Notice the sensations in your knee and in your thigh. Return to the starting position, still initiating the movement from the lateral side of the left knee.

Now rub the *inside* (medial area) of the left knee and place your attention there as you initiate a movement of the knee toward the foot from the inside of your knee. Once again, notice the different sensations in your leg, thigh, and ankle as the inside of the left knee initiates the movement toward the foot. Return the knee to the starting position, still initiating from the inside area of the left knee.

Each movement has been in the same direction, but the muscles organize and function slightly differently when the movement is initiated from a slightly different place.

Injury, misuse, and poor postural alignment can limit range of motion and strain overused and ineffective movement patterns. When we initiate movement from various places, we are offering our muscles and nervous system new options for organization and movement, thus freeing the body from restrictive, and often painful, patterning.

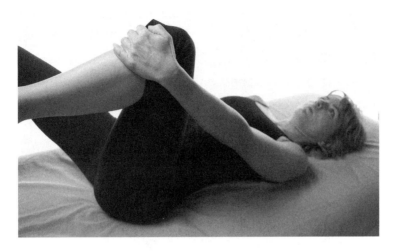

Fig. 4.12. Rub front of knee

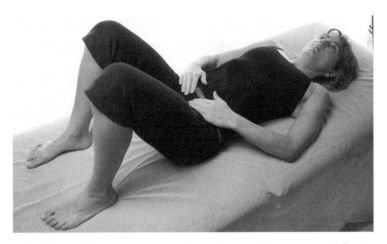

Fig. 4.13. Initiate movement from front of knee toward foot

※ ※ ※

Isometric Releases and Exercises for Femur Alignment (for Cellulite, Pain in the Hip Socket, or Traveler's Hip)

Alignment of the femur is important for establishing a sense of foundation and security in your walk, for getting your feet underneath you, and being able to walk with feet parallel.

These isometric exercises balance and cue the deep muscles that support proper alignment of the femur for weight transfer and optimal forward and rotational movement. The exercises also can help to relieve pain in the hip socket. As a side note, proper alignment of the femur helps the muscles of the hip and thigh to work more efficiently, which can help to eliminate cellulite.

This is a great release technique for frequent flyers tending to hold or stabilize their weight in one hip while sitting on long flights. I have often used this isometric exercise to release tension or pain in my hip after, or even during, a flight. Anyone who frequently sits for long periods of time or sits with one leg crossed over the other can benefit from this release.

Remember: Always begin an isometric exercise in the preferred and comfortable position. Apply light resistance for seven to ten seconds as you try to move out of the comfortable position. After releasing the resistance, use your hand to passively *move the thigh bone in the direction that you were attempting to go during the isometric. By "passively" I mean use your hand, not the muscles of the upper leg, to move the femur. Also keep in mind that the muscles that you are accessing here might be smaller and weaker than the ones you have normally been using, so slight, small movements assist these muscles to strengthen and reeducate.*

PREPARATION: ASSESSING FEMUR ALIGNMENT ,,,

➤ To determine the alignment of your femur, look at your thighs while sitting or standing. Note the roundness of their front surface. If you tend to rotate your thigh externally (out to the side), the thigh will appear flatter. If you tend to rotate your thigh internally (in toward the midline of your body), the thigh will appear rounder. First compare the thighs: does one look flatter or one rounder?

Next, while sitting, rock one knee and thigh toward the midline of your body and then out to the side of your body. Notice if internal or external rotation feels more comfortable for you. Use your hands to slightly exaggerate the internal or external rotation preference (Figures 4.14 and 4.15).

Perhaps one thigh will prefer one direction while the other prefers the opposite direction. If there is resistance or pain in either direction or in the hip socket, use the following isometric exercises to balance the muscles around the joint and open movement potential.

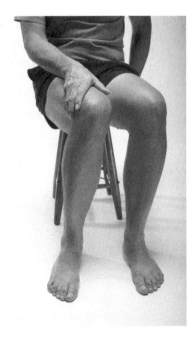

Fig. 4.14. Check for internal preference

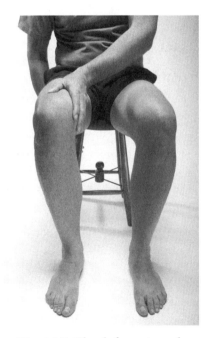

Fig. 4.15. Check for external preference

RELEASE FOR EXTERNAL ROTATION OF THE FEMUR (FLAT THIGH)⁗⁗⁗⁗

➤ If the thigh appears flatter and prefers to move *away* from the midline of the body, rotate the thigh and knee away from the midline into its preference. Place your opposite hand along the inside of your knee to create resistance to midline movement (Figure 4.16).

Imagine that you are initiating movement to internally rotate the thigh toward the other leg (midline of the body). Initiate the rotational movement from the top of the thigh bone in the hip socket to bring the knee toward midline. The resisting hand blocks the actual movement for ten seconds and then supports a follow-through movement toward the midline (Figure 4.17).

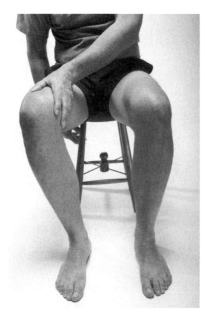

Fig. 4.16. Hand resists internal rotation

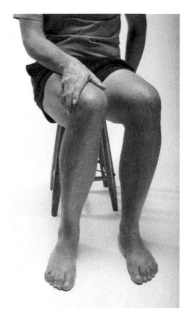

Fig. 4.17. Passively move thigh internally

RELEASE FOR INTERNAL ROTATION OF THE FEMUR (ROUND THIGH)‚‚‚‚‚‚‚‚‚‚

➤ If the thigh appears rounder and prefers to move *toward* the midline of the body, rotate the thigh and knee toward the midline into its preference. Place your opposite hand along the outside of your knee to create resistance to lateral movement (Figure 4.18).

Imagine that you are initiating a lateral movement within the hip socket to rotate the thigh away from midline. Initiate movement from the top of the femur in the hip socket to externally rotate the thigh. The resisting hand blocks the external movement for ten seconds and then supports the thigh as the leg moves laterally to follow through and complete the attempted movement (Figure 4.19).

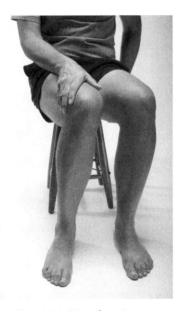

Fig. 4.18. Hand resists external rotation

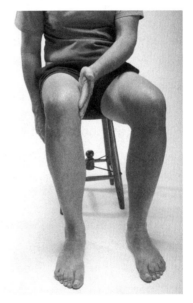

Fig. 4.19. Passively complete movement

STRENGTHENING ISOMETRIC FOR EXTERNAL ROTATION
OF THE FEMUR (FLAT THIGH)

If you are able to cross your ankle over your opposite knee, try this isometric exercise for alignment and strengthening of the small muscles around the head of the femur.

If your thigh feels more comfortable rotating away from the midline of your body and appears flatter when you are sitting, use this isometric exercise for external rotation.

➤ Sitting, cross the ankle of the externally rotated leg onto the knee of the opposite leg. Note how this position exaggerates the external rotation. Then place your opposite hand on the knee of the rotated leg. You will use this hand to create a very small amount of resistance (Figure 4.20).

With your focus on the top of the femur, where it sits in the hip socket, imagine that you are initiating a small rotational movement of the femur and knee toward the midline of your body. Then actually slowly initiate a small, slow movement from the top of the femur in the hip socket to rotate the femur toward the center (medially). Your knee will attempt to move toward the opposite shoulder against the slight resistance from the pressure of your hand. Keep the hand's resistance to a minimum, while you maintain your focus and the initiation of the movement at the top of the femur in the hip socket.

If you initiate the movement from the knee or with too much power, you will probably override the cueing that needs to begin at the hip socket, and will end up reinforcing the old movement pattern.

After ten seconds of the attempted movement, stop resisting it, and passively move the thigh and knee to complete the attempted movement (Figure 4.21).

If you're unable to cross your ankle over your opposite knee, the two exercises immediately above will work just as well.

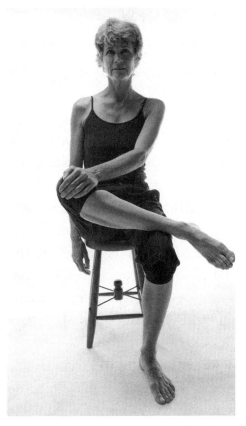

Fig. 4.20. Pressure against hand to rotate femur internally

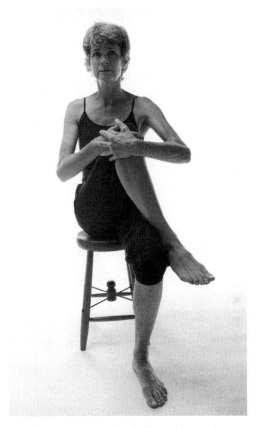

Fig. 4.21. Passive follow-through of attempted movement

STRENGTHENING ISOMETRIC FOR INTERNAL ROTATION OF THE FEMUR (ROUND THIGH)

For internal rotation of the femur, the thigh will appear rounded and may slightly resist external rotation.

➤ Sit and rest the ankle of the internally rotated (affected) side on the opposite knee. With your opposite hand, reach across to lift and support the knee in the position raised toward midline. This hand will be used to give a slight amount of resistance during the isometric exercise (Figure 4.22).

Focus on the top of the femur of the affected (raised) leg and imagine the femur rotating out to the side (laterally). Then slowly initiate a movement from the top of the femur to laterally rotate the femur in the hip socket. This will cause the knee to attempt to move downward into the initially supporting, and now resisting, hand. Keep the resistance to a minimum and maintain your focus and initiation of the movement at the top of the femur where it fits into the hip socket.

If you initiate the movement from the knee or with too much power, you will probably override the necessary cueing at the hip socket and will end up reinforcing the old movement pattern.

After ten seconds, release the resistance and passively move the thigh and knee with your hand to complete the attempted movement (Figure 4.23).

If you're unable to cross your ankle over your opposite knee, you may use the Releases for External and Internal Rotation, above, in this section.

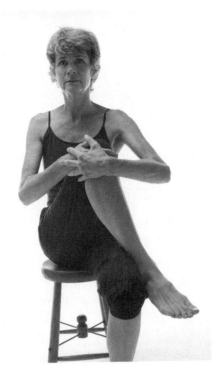

Fig. 4.22. Pressure against hand to externally rotate femur

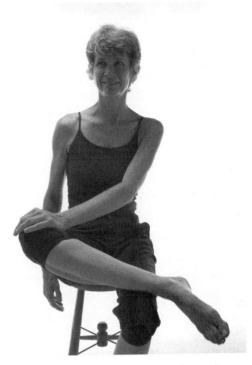

Fig. 4.23. Passive follow-through of attempted movement

CHAPTER 5

Hamstrings and Calves

The muscles at the back of the legs can become very tight and hold a lot of tension. Many cases of plantar fasciitis of the foot originate in the tension patterns of the calves and hamstrings (muscles at the back of the thigh). The standard treatment usually involves stretching the muscles of the back of the legs.

I recommend that you do these very simple releases before stretching. These releases, which I learned from an Australian Ortho-Bionomy practitioner who works with athletes, are amazingly effective for releasing leg tensions. Try doing one leg and then stand and walk, so you can compare the difference between the two legs.

Do this release either sitting on the edge of a chair or standing with your foot or knee resting on a stool. Use whichever position helps you to feel more comfortable.

➤ Place your hand on your calf or hamstring and simply move the tissue down toward your foot and then up toward your hips. Then move and hold for ten to thirty seconds in whichever direction feels more comfortable to you. If both directions feel comfortable then move in the direction that the tissue moves most easily.

Next, move the tissue toward the other leg and then away from it. Once again, choose the more comfortable position for the hamstring muscles or tissue of your calf and hold for ten to thirty seconds (Figure 5.1).

You might also try diagonal movements, once again holding in the more comfortable direction.

Remember that you don't have to use much pressure; just gently push the skin and tissue in the direction it goes most easily. This simple release can be applied anywhere there is tension stored in the tissue.

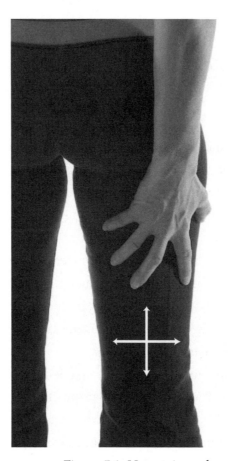

Figure 5.1. Hamstring release

CHAPTER 6

Knee

The knee functions to create stability while bearing weight and supporting movement. This is accomplished mainly through alignment of the femur with the tibia and the complex support structure of ligaments, tendons, and cartilage. As the joint in the middle of the leg, the knee mediates movement and weight-bearing from the hip above, and compression and movement from the ankle and foot below.

Knee tension may be a result of a femur rotation, or misaligned patterning in the hip, ankle or foot, the walking pattern, or in the sacroiliac joint. If knee tension continues after the releases, you may need to try the "Initiating Movement from Different Places" awareness exercise in Chapter 4, the release positions for rotation of the hip (Chapter 3), the releases for the ankle (Chapter 7) and the foot (Chapter 8), and femur rotation isometrics (Chapter 4). Follow these up with the "Repatterning Your Walk" exercises in Chapter 9; the "Teenage Telephone Talk" to release the sacroiliac joint in Chapter 3; and "Supine Kicking" in Chapter 17 to exercise the sacroiliac joint.

Anatomy of the Knee

The bones that comprise the knee joint are the thigh bone (femur), the shin bone (tibia), and the kneecap (patella). See Figure 6.1. There is another lower leg bone outside (lateral to) the tibia called the fibula. The fibula connects only with the other lower leg bone, not with the thigh bone. The fibula acts as a type of flying buttress to support the lower leg. Its support for the knee is indirect, but important.

Important:

Always release the kneecap before using any of the other release positions for the knee.

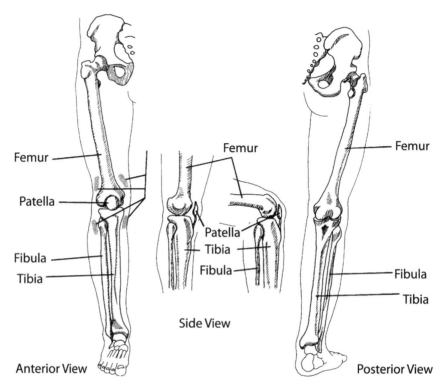

Fig. 6.1. Knee

Releases for the Knee

KNEECAP RELEASE ///

➤ Sit in a relaxed position with the legs straight out but not locked. Gently hold the kneecap (patella) between your thumb and fingertips.

Gently push the patella medial (toward the other leg) and then lateral (to the outside), noting any directional preference or resistance to movement. Move the kneecap to the direction of ease and preference and hold for ten to thirty seconds (Figures 6.2 and 6.3).

Release and recheck the kneecap for increased movement range in both directions. (If the patella does not move easily in any direction, you may need to recline slightly to relax it.)

Next move the patella down toward the foot and then up toward the head, once again assessing for ease of movement and comfort. Move in the direction of ease and hold for ten to thirty seconds (Figures 6.4 and 6.5).

Then check for patella movement along the four corner diagonals—up and out and down and in, up and in and down and out (Figures 6.6 and 6.7). Release and recheck for increased movement range in all four directions.

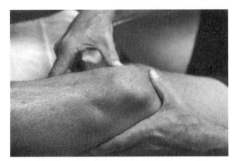 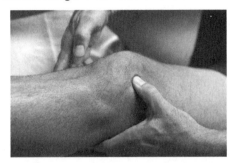

Figs. 6.2 and 6.3. Push patella side to side

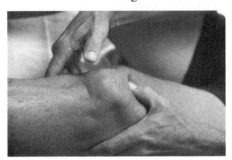 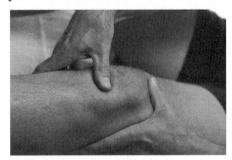

Figs. 6.4 and 6.5. Push patella down and up

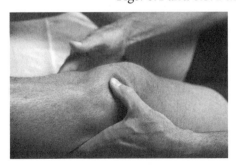 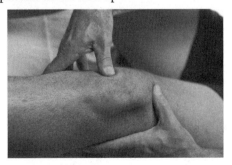

Figs. 6.6 and 6.7. Push patella diagonally

MASTER KNEE RELEASE POSITION //

The Master Knee Release position is for tender points on the medial side (inside) of the knee, just above and below the head of the tibia where it meets the lower femur (Figure 6.8). Position the knee in such a way that allows the tender points to be cradled within a "curve."

➤ Bend the knee and rest the ankle on the opposite knee. You can lightly rest your finger on the tender point to monitor it for softening and/or pulsation. You may do this positioning either sitting or while lying on your back, whichever is more comfortable. Place your hand on your heel and gently torque the heel of the foot toward the knee.

To fine-tune the position to the specific point that is tender, experiment with bending the knee more or less and lifting the ankle slightly until you attain maximum softening or a pulsation release at the tender point.

You will know when you have the best release position because the tenderness will be greatly reduced, the tissue will have softened, and you may feel a slight pulsation at the point that was sore.

When you have determined the best position, slowly compress from the torqued heel up toward the knee, sensing for pulsation or release at the point. Hold in this position for ten to thirty seconds. Slowly come out of the position so as not to reintroduce the holding pattern (Figure 6.9).

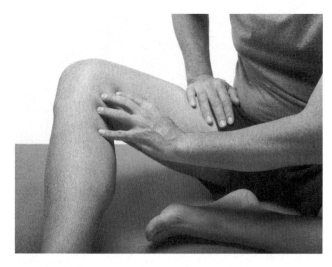

Fig. 6.8. Check for tender points

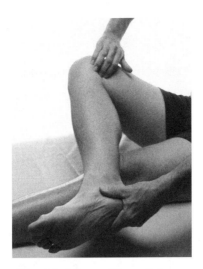

Fig. 6.9. Master Knee Release

RELEASING PAIN AND TENDERNESS
ON THE OUTSIDE (LATERAL SIDE) OF THE KNEE ,,,

➤ To release tender points on the lateral side of the knee, sit on the floor or bed, bend your knee, and place your foot on the bed or floor. Bring the foot slightly out to the side (lateral from midline) and let the knee fall slightly toward midline. Grasp the top of the knee and gently pull the skin and under-lying tissue toward the tender point at the side of the knee (Figure 6.10).

This positioning may also release tender points behind and below the head of the fibula, or you can try the alternative positioning below.

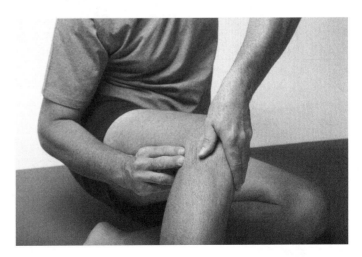

Fig. 6.10. Side of knee release

RELEASING THE FIBULA

➤ To release tender points behind (posterior to) or below (inferior to) the head of the fibula (the bone on the outside of the lower leg), sit on the floor or bed and bend the knee.

If—and only if—this is comfortable for you, bring your foot out to the side toward your hip, letting your knee drop medially toward the bed. Grasp and gently torque the heel back toward the fibula, sensing for softening or pulsing at the tender points below or behind the head of the fibula (Figure 6.11).

If comfortable, hold the position for ten to thirty seconds, then release.

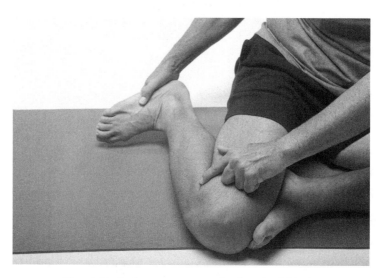

Fig. 6.11. Release position for head of fibula

ALTERNATIVE FIBULA RELEASE

➤ You may also release the fibula with a more subtle technique. Sitting so that you can contact the head of the fibula bone, gently push the head of the fibula toward the front of the leg and back, noting the most comfortable preference.

With your other hand contact the lower head of the fibula at the malleolus (lateral bone of the ankle). Gently push this part of the fibula toward the front of the ankle and back, noting the comfortable preference.

Hold both ends of the fibula in their respective preferred positions for ten to sixty seconds or until you feel the fibula begin to subtly rebound (Figure 6.12).

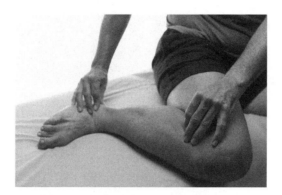

Fig. 6.12. Fibula release

%% %% %%

Movement Exercises for the Knee

KNEE ROCKING FOR INTEGRATION ,,

After the knee releases, reestablish a balanced movement relationship among the hip, knee, ankle, and foot. I cannot overemphasize how important gentle movement is to open up the functioning, balance, and reintegration of an area. This exercise allows the nervous system to recalibrate and integrate balanced movement among all the muscles of the hip, leg, and ankle for optimum functioning. It is incredibly effective any time you have knee discomfort. This exercise can be done gently and slowly even after surgery.

➤ Lie on your back with your knees bent and your feet on the floor or bed. Line up your feet with your hips and knees.

Then initiate movement from your knees to slowly rock them side to side within your range of comfort. Notice the steady, balanced movement in the knees, hips, ankles, and feet (Figures 6.13 and 6.14). You can also do this exercise while sitting.

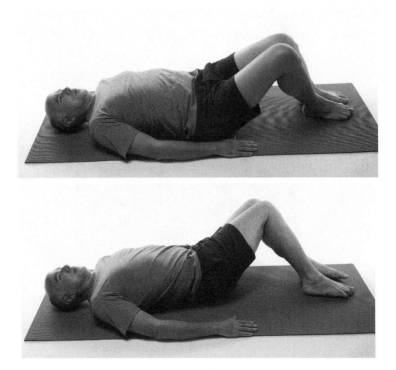

Figs. 6.13 and 6.14. Rock knees side to side

KNEE CIRCLES TO STRENGTHEN HEALTHY KNEES ///

Be sure to track your comfort in this exercise. If you experience pain with the positioning or movement, try some of the knee releases first.

➤ Stand with your knees together, slightly bent. Place your hands on your knees and slowly draw circles parallel to the floor, keeping your knees together. Move your knees to the right side and then to the back. Complete the circular motion by moving the knees to the left side and again to the front (Figures 6.15 to 6.18).

Note any places in the circle where you feel discomfort or tension in the knees. Move into a position directly *across* the circle from the discomfort and hold for five to thirty seconds.

Recheck by moving your knees in circles in both directions. If there is still discomfort, move to a position in the circle just *before* the discomfort and hold the position for five to twenty seconds.

Then circle your knees again and recheck for comfort.

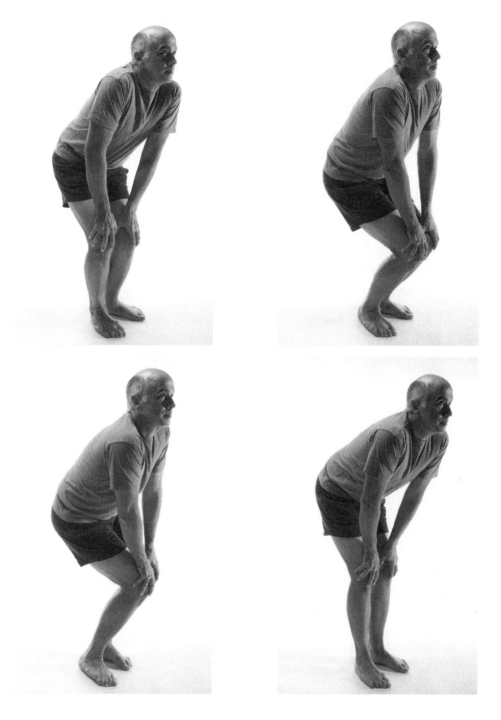

Figs. 6.15 to 6.18. Knee Circles

❉ ❉ ❉

CHAPTER 7

Ankle

Treating a Sprain

Years ago, while on a camping trip with my family in the magnificent redwood trees of northern California, we climbed up on a fallen giant sequoia to sit and take some photographs. As I jumped down I fell, twisting and seriously spraining my ankle. Immediately I sat down exactly where I fell and placed my hands ever so lightly on my ankle. I encouraged the family to go on ahead and start the picnic lunch, assuring them I would be okay and would come join them soon.

With my hands barely touching my ankle, I sensed the shock to the area and the waves of pain. I was patient and attentive the way I would be with a crying child who may have just fallen from her bike. When that first wave of dismay over the injury passed, I let my fingers gently rest on the skin, quietly noting tiny movement patterns. As my ankle began to trust the contact, I let my fingers follow the slight movements felt just at skin level. I followed the skin movement in one direction until it stopped and then checked to see if there was a right- or left-turn preference, always choosing the direction of least resistance. Once I felt that the skin was willing to move in all directions easily, I moved my attention to the layer of tissue below the skin, again slowly following the tissue preferences of movement. As that layer felt attuned to, it slowly unwound its tissue holding patterns. I worked with each layer of tissue until eventually I was able to work with the muscle layer, once again slowly following the movement patterns—moving in one direction until I reached a stopping point and then making a right or left turn in the direction of least resistance.

Next, I worked with the joint itself. I let the patterns of release within the muscles lead me into the movement preferences of the joint. In just twenty minutes I was able to get up and walk to join my family for lunch. The ankle was virtually pain-free as long as I walked on the even-surfaced concrete paths. I experienced a little pain if I tried to walk on the wood chips. The tiny intrinsic muscles of my ankle were still healing and weren't quite ready to accommodate the uneven surface.

After lunch my ankle felt pretty good as we hiked to the van for the three-hour drive back to the Bay Area. At home, as I got out and stepped down, a slight soreness reminded me that I had injured myself, but I was surprised to notice that there was no swelling. I sat down again and repeated the sequence as before, following the tissue movement patterns through the tissue layers to the muscle and into the joint. The next morning I still had no swelling, no bruising, and no tenderness at all.

Once again, the value of this work to assist in the self-healing capacity of the body was confirmed for me.

Anatomy of the Ankle

The lower heads of the lower leg bones (tibia and fibula) widen to meet and snugly fit around the talus bone of the foot, forming the ankle joint. The bump on the inside of the ankle is actually the lower head of the tibia widening out to cradle the talus bone of the foot. This tibia bump on the inside of the ankle is called the medial malleolus. The bump on the outside of the ankle is the lower head of the fibula bone. This fibula bump is called the lateral malleolus (Figure 7.1).

These two leg bones and the surrounding ligaments and muscles provide stability for the flexibility of the talus bone of the foot. The top of the talus bone is shaped like a saddle, and the inner surfaces of the tibia and fibula meet it in such a way as to offer support and flexibility so that the leg rides and glides over the talus bone when we walk.

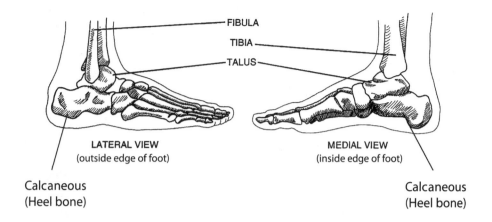

Fig. 7.1. Ankle

Releases for the Ankle

OPPOSITE SIDE OF THE CIRCLE //

➤ Sit and hold your ankle in your lap, slowly rotating your foot to circle the ankle. Note any restrictions to the movement or areas of discomfort. If there are any, gently move the ankle directly across the circle to the area opposite the restriction or discomfort. Support the ankle in this position and add gentle compression toward the joint for about ten to thirty seconds (Figures 7.2 to 7.6).

Or, move the ankle to a place just before the discomfort or glitch, holding in that position and applying comfortable compression toward the joint for five to thirty seconds.

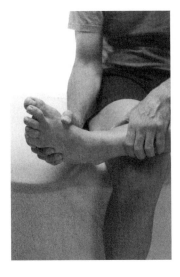
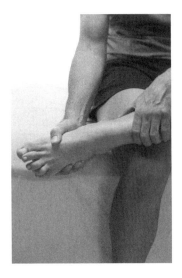
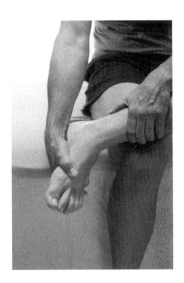

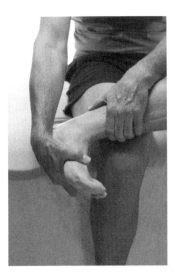
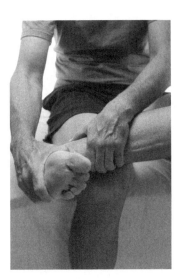

Figs. 7.2 to 7.6. Ankle rotations

INJURED ANKLE RELEASE //

➤ Let your ankle tell its story. Listen to how it wants to be touched, held, and the specific ways it wants to be moved. Just listening and attending to the tissue can help us reconnect with the injured part and remind us that, with care and attention, injuries can heal.

When working with any recently injured area, it is important to use the lightest touch. Think of turning a fine-tuning dial that regulates the amount of pressure and contact to address any area in the most comfortable way.

This slow, subtle movement encourages the tissue to release any trauma or shock and helps to reestablish balance in the tissue and circulation around the joints.

Gently place your hands or fingertips on the sprained or painful ankle. Slowly feel for the direction of preferred skin movement and using your fingertips, follow the movement preferences of the skin tissue. These sensations may be subtle, but essentially you are following the tissue in one direction until it stops. Then you make a right or a left turn to feel which direction is preferred, and follow it that way.

Once the skin has released restrictions of its movement, follow the movement preferences of the tissue layer under the skin. After the underlying tissue has begun to release its restrictions, slowly and gently support and follow the tiny movements inherent at the joints, as I describe in the first section of this chapter (Figures 7.7 to 7.9).

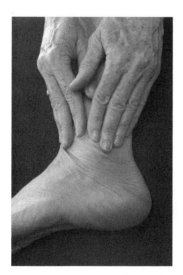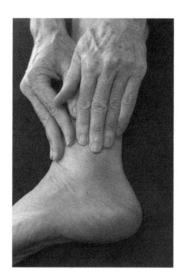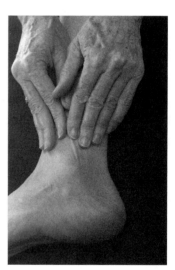

Figs. 7.7 to 7.9. Follow movement preference of tissue

Movement Exercises for the Ankle

FLEXION/EXTENSION OF THE ANKLE ,,

Many of us walk with our toes continuously flexed and our ankles barely moving. This exercise encourages us to work our ankles more and gives the smaller muscles connecting to our toes a rest. Resting the toes in this manner will benefit our shoulders as well, since this area of the toes reflexes to the shoulders.

➤ Sit with legs outstretched and bend at the ankle so that the upper foot flexes back toward the leg. For some, the toes may be quite involved in initiating the movement. If that is true for you, then try to do this without activating the toes, keeping them relaxed and neutral, with the movement initiating in the ankle (Figures 7.10 and 7.11).

Experiment to see if it is easier to do this movement with one ankle than with the other. Practice with both ankles until you can do both with the same ease. It may help if you consciously think about allowing your heel to extend away from your leg as you bend at the ankle.

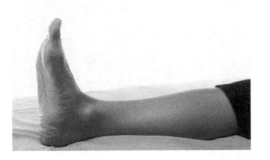 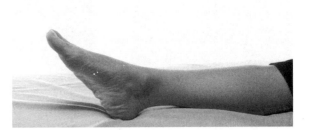

Figs. 7.10 and 7.11. Flexion and extension of the ankle

STRENGTHENING THE ANKLE
WITH AN ISOTONIC EXERCISE *,,*

(See "Isometric and Isotonic Movements" in Chapter 1)

A "turned" or sprained ankle can overstretch the muscles on the side of the ankle, creating an imbalance in muscle strength. Often there is more weakness or lack of smooth movement when rolling the foot toward the outside of the leg (eversion) than when rolling the foot toward the other leg (inversion). Balancing the muscle strength in both directions with this isotonic exercise tends to strengthen the ankle and support alignment through the leg and hip.

This exercise may be done sitting, lying, or standing on one leg.

➤ Observe your foot as you roll the sole of the foot toward the medial line (invert) and toward the outside of the leg (evert). Are you able to make these movements evenly and smoothly in each direction? Which direction feels more comfortable to you (Figures 7.12 and 7.13)?

Now sit and hold the ankle with your hand in its comfortable position, so you can provide slight resistance to movement. Begin to roll the side of the foot toward the opposite direction while your hand offers some resistance (Figures 7.14 and 7.15) yet still allows the ankle to move slowly.

Begin with only a very slight resistance. As you become more familiar with the movement, add a bit more resistance, which strengthens the ankle muscles. Too much resistance overpowers the small intrinsic muscles that you are attempting to strengthen, so remember to just give enough that the muscles need to work a little but don't have to strain.

If this movement is unfamiliar and/or very difficult to do, then slowly take the foot passively (i.e., move it with your hands) through the movement first. Then try it with the ankle muscles moving it.

You may repeat this exercise a few times, but rest if the muscles feel tired. When you over-tire muscles that you are attempting to strengthen, you may well revert to your old pattern.

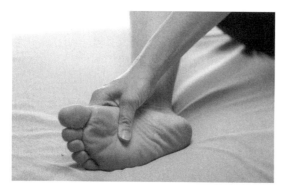

Fig. 7.12. Ankle inversion

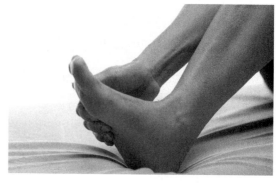

Fig. 7.13. Ankle eversion

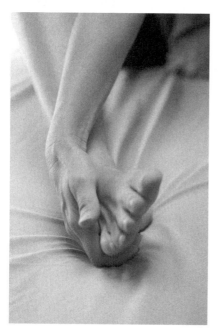

Fig. 7.14. Side of foot presses and moves against hand to strengthen ankle

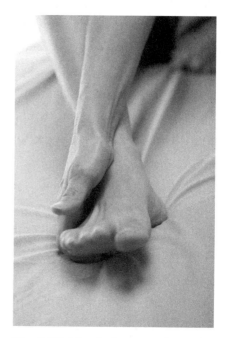

Fig. 7.15. Hand gives steady pressure, allowing foot to straighten

※ ※ ※

CHAPTER 8

Foot

As bipedal creatures, our feet literally form the foundation upon which we physically stand. Phrases like "having your feet firmly planted" and "standing on your own two feet" embody the ideas of foundation, stable base, groundedness, and connection with the earth. Yet the feet are so much more than a stable, static, grounded base. When you consider the complexity of walking, jumping, or running—all variations of throwing our weight forward and catching ourselves with each step—it's amazing how the body balances on such relatively small and flexible structures. I invite you to take time to explore and celebrate the wonder of your feet as you work with the release positions.

Anatomy of the Foot

The foot is a wonderful design. It all comes down to twenty-six small bones that support, stabilize, and absorb the shock of our weight shifting as we move. Muscles and ligaments bind these small bones together yet allow flexibility in the joints.

The lower leg bones nestle and rock on the saddle-like top of the talus bone, creating the ankle joint. When standing, the weight is transferred down through the shin bone (tibia) to the talus, then simultaneously back through the heel bone (calcaneous), and forward through the other bones of the feet, creating a stable triangular base.

Just forward of the talus and the calcaneous are seven bones, collectively referred to as the tarsals. Moving down the foot, next are the five long metatarsal bones, which in turn connect to the bones of our toes, the phalanges (Figure 8.1).

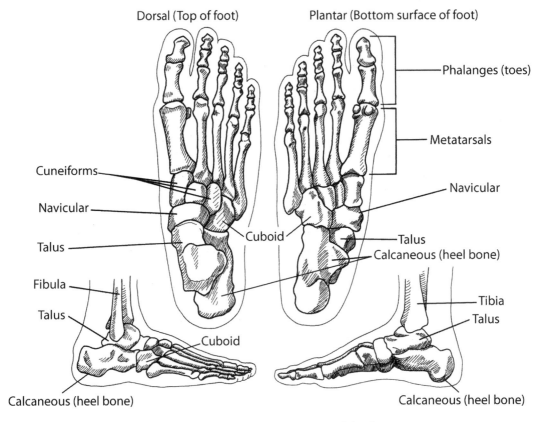

Fig. 8.1. Bones of the foot

Healing the Trauma of a Broken Foot

A dear young woman who had broken many of the bones in her foot came to the office for regular sessions. The trauma of the injury and fear about medical intervention kept her from considering surgery. She had learned to be compassionate with herself and had been creatively making her own shoes as a way to create comfort and support for her foot.

In our sessions together, we began by exploring the ways her foot had created safety and functionality for itself while healing. I used general releases in which I curved around the tender points and then gently added compression toward the joints.

Gradually, as greater flexibility returned to her foot, she felt empowered to work with a local shoemaker who built shoes that comfortably supported and exercised her foot. These shoes exercised her foot in the same way that the Ortho-Bionomy sessions had affirmed and restored her flexibility. So often injury, trauma, and pain can seem to immobilize us, but gentle, slow, and exploratory attention and perseverance can have empowering and rewarding results, even after years of discomfort.

Releases for the Foot

These positional release techniques increase the foot's flexibility. Remember to move slowly as you explore the positions. Moving too quickly may result in skipping over the position of optimum release. Give yourself an opportunity to fully feel and affirm your comfort.

GENERAL CURVING AROUND THE SORE POINTS,,

➤ Feel around your foot for tender points. Then gently bend the foot in such a way as to comfortably create a "curve" or a "cave" around the tender point. Just a small insinuation of a cave can be enough.

Then add compression toward the point or toward the joint. Hold the compression for ten to thirty seconds or until you feel a shift or release (Figures 8.2 and 8.3).

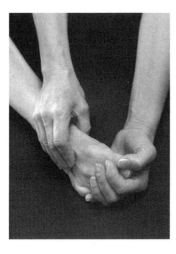
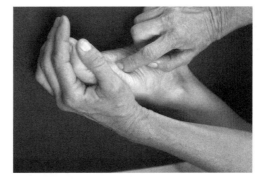

Figs. 8.2 and 8.3. Curling around sore points

EXPLORING THE LONG BONES OF THE FOOT ///

➤ Explore between the metatarsals, the long bones in the feet that attach to the toes. Do you sense free movement between these bones, or do they feel tightly connected? If there is tightness between two of them, compress them together in the direction of the tension and hold for a few seconds. Then recheck to see if movement has increased (Figures 8.4 to 8.6).

If there is general tension throughout all the metatarsals, then compress all of them by grasping across the top of the foot and squeezing the sides of the foot together for ten to thirty seconds.

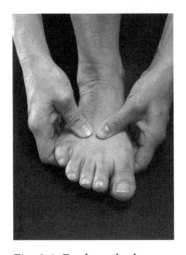

Fig. 8.4. Explore the long bones of the foot

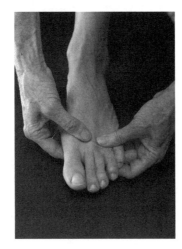

Fig. 8.5. Squeeze the metatarsals together

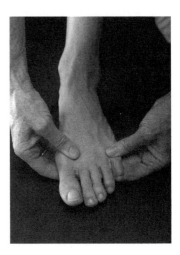

Fig. 8.6. Pull metatarsals apart

METATARSAL RELEASE ///

➤ Perhaps it feels as if one metatarsal is lower and the adjacent one is higher. Exaggerate this positioning slightly by pushing the lower one down and the higher one up, then compress them together and hold for a few seconds. Then separate and recheck for greater ease of movement and less tension (Figures 8.7 and 8.8).

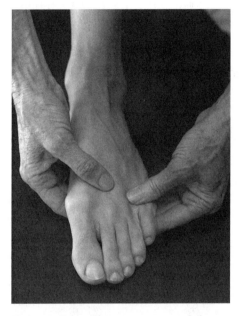

Fig. 8.7. Press lower metatarsal down and squeeze metatarsals together

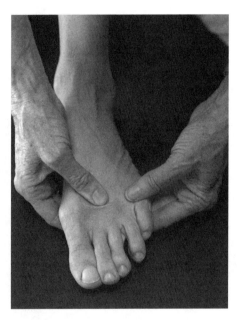

Fig. 8.8. Pull metatarsals apart

DROPPED METATARSAL RELEASE //

➤ Sometimes the head of a metatarsal (where it meets the toe) has dropped down toward the sole of the foot. This can be assessed by feeling for a tender point or bump under the ball of the foot.

If you find a dropped metatarsal, simply lift the corresponding toe upward at the tip and gently compress the toe back toward where it meets the foot. This will slightly exaggerate the bump on the bottom of the foot even more (Figure 8.9).

Hold for a minute and then release out of the compressed position by slowly pulling out the toe, giving it a gentle stretch (Figure 8.10).

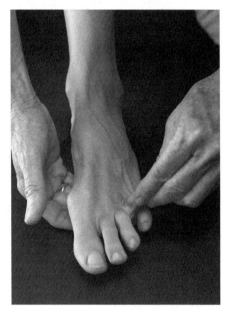

Fig. 8.9. Lift toe and push down to exaggerate dropped metatarsal

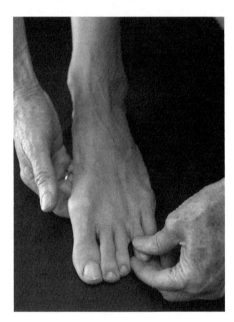

Fig. 8.10. Stretch toe after release

BIG TOE RELEASE //

This release for the big toe also helps to reflexively release tensions in the neck.

➤ Explore the area where the big toe attaches to the foot, especially between the big toe and the second toe. If there is tenderness at the base of the big toe, rotate the toe toward the point of tension and compress the toe into the foot. Hold the compression for a few seconds. Then gently and slowly pull on the toe to stretch and lengthen as you release the compression. Recheck the point again to see if the tenderness has cleared (Figures 8.11 and 8.12).

If you have sore bunions, see Chapter 18.

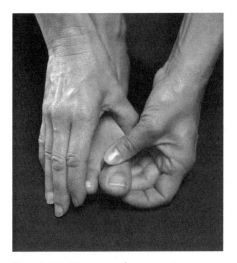

Fig. 8.11. Big toe release point

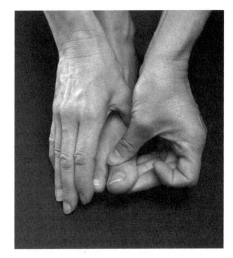

Fig. 8.12. Rotate big toe
and compress

%, %, %,

CHAPTER 9

Walking

Walking is an act of transferring weight and is accomplished through five springs and the support of the three arches. By sensing the direct contact between our feet and the ground and sensing the pattern of correct movement, we can create a more balanced and coherent pattern of walking, one that generates and supports better alignment throughout the legs, knees and hips.

Three Arches of the Foot

There are three functional arches to the foot: the lateral, medial, and transverse (Figure 9.1). The lateral (outside) arch consists of the heel bone (calcaneous), the cuboid, and the fourth and fifth toes and the long bones that connect to them (metatarsals). It absorbs, supports, and carries the body weight forward along the outside edge of the foot during walking.

The medial (inside) longitudinal arch is the one we usually think about when we buy arch supports. It provides the power to push off to take the next step. It consists of the first, second, and third toes; the long bones that connect to them (metatarsals); and the talus, the navicular, and the cuneiforms.

The transverse arch offers flexibility, stability, and shock-absorber support to the foot. It consists of the three cuneiforms, the cuboid, and the five metatarsals.

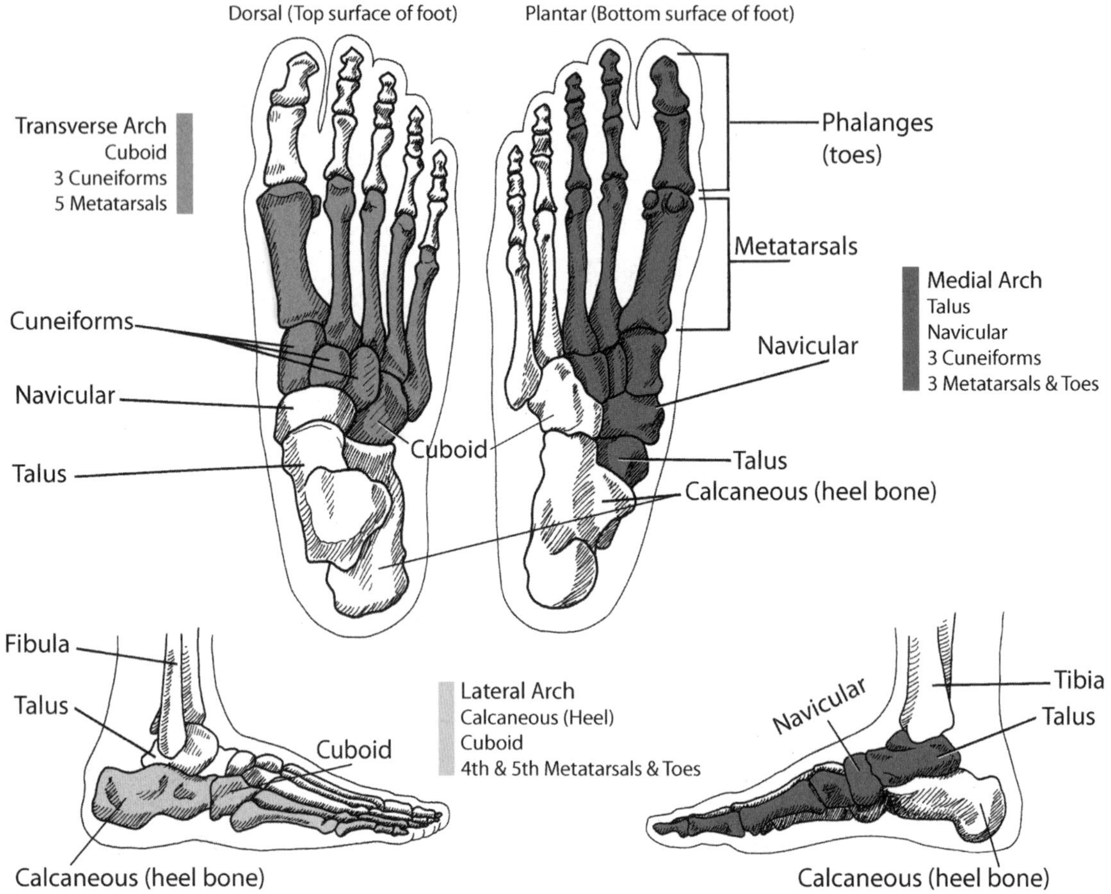

Fig. 9.1. Three arches of the foot

Five Springs of the Foot

- First Spring: The first spring is very subtle to feel and most of the time we are moving too fast to notice it at all. Yet this tiny action begins to direct the weight slightly toward the outside (lateral) arch of the foot. Notice as your weight comes down on the heel bone the slight natural tendency to roll the weight over to the outside of this bone.
- Second Spring: Once the weight is transferred to the outside of the heel, it continues rolling down the outside (lateral aspect) of our foot along the lateral longitudinal line toward the base of the little toe, along the lateral arch.

- Third Spring: At the third spring, this movement and weight is then transferred from the base of the little toe across the metatarsal bones to the base of the big toe. This third spring is held in check by the transverse arch of the foot (cuboid, cuneiform, and metatarsal bones).

- Fourth Spring: Next, the weight shifts from the base of the big toe onto the big toe itself. This movement connects us to the medial (inside) longitudinal arch and gives us the maximum amount of support.

- Fifth Spring: Drawing on a maximum amount of support of the medial (inner) longitudinal arch and the maximum extension of the big toe, we use this support and extension as a spring to push off the foot.

REPATTERNING YOUR WALK ,,

➤ Sitting or standing with most of your weight resting on one foot, slowly trace the movement of weight along the five springs of your other foot. Transfer weight on your heel to the outside of the heel, down the outside of the foot to the base of the little toe. Then shift the weight across to the base of the big toe and sense the support of the medial (inside) longitudinal arch. Feel this support and the extension of the big toe creating the impulse and propulsion for the push-off (Figure 9.2).

Try slowly repeating this patterning movement a few times on one foot, then on the other. When you can stay with sensing the movement pattern, try the next exercise, "Slow-Motion Walking."

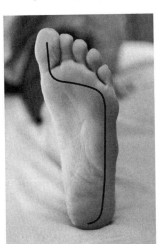

Remember any exercise of reeducation or repatterning offers the body an option, an alternative. Offer the option frequently, perhaps two to three times daily, yet give the body a chance to integrate the new sensory information at its own pace.

Fig. 9.2. Sequence of foot contact

SLOW-MOTION WALKING

➤ Practice slow-motion walking. Walk slowly enough to sense the movement from the heel to the outside of the foot, down to the base of the little toe, across to the base of the big toe, and finally on to the big toe itself for the final push-off.

Sense the support of the three arches and the weight transfer that happens at the five springs of the feet.

※ ※ ※

III. Inspiration and Expression—Upper Body

֍ ֍ ֍

The Heart of the Matter

The area of the heart is associated with feelings of love, tenderness, and compassion. When we consider these qualities, we generally think in terms of having these feelings for others. Yet maintaining this same regard for oneself creates an attitude of acceptance and non-judgment that allows us to surrender to our experience and our own sense of relaxation.

Recently, I was working with a woman who had pain in her upper back. A student of Ortho-Bionomy herself, she had tried many of the positions of release but complained that it was difficult to get compression where she needed it. I suggested that maybe she didn't need compression. Perhaps she could just find the best position of release and then surrender to her heart.

The offering of compassionate acceptance for oneself often brings release when nothing else seems to work. A calm heart offers a resting place where we can give up our fears, fixed attitudes, and pain, and renew our spirit. Creating a space of quiet repose allows us to shift our mood and bring our attention to an internal sense of relaxation and restfulness.

Accessing Self-Compassion in the Moment of Discomfort

When we can access self-compassion and the calm neutral witness right in the moment of discomfort and pain, we can be more present with our experience. This helps us notice and not react to the pain but to work with ourselves in a clear and useful way. We can place our frustration aside just for the moment and begin to experiment to see if there is one small thing that will bring us more comfort.

For example, right now I feel a pain in my upper spine as I sit here at the computer. I notice an annoyance to this ache and a bit of tension on the left side. I begin to bring my attention into the sensation and explore this pain with curiosity. I note that there is also a feeling of tiredness in my spine on the left. By slowly side-bending a tiny bit to the right, I notice that my annoyance is gone, and the sensation at my spine has shifted to numbness. If I add a slight right rotation to the side-bending position, I notice that the numbness, tension, and pain are gone. I let myself rest in this comfort for a moment or two. Now, as I shift back to a centered neutral position, I notice a sense of relief.

By attending to the body in the moment, we can discover the positions that bring a sense of ease. We can recognize that just by directing our compassionate neutral attention to the sensations of the moment, we allow our sensation to direct us toward comfort.

Creating tender compassion for your direct sensory experience helps you to release and surrender your attitudes, fears, and discomfort and to begin to notice the subtle proximity of ease and well-being. As we practice this way of being with ourselves we are cultivating new habits to replace old non-useful tendencies to create or reinforce tension patterns in expectation or fear of pain. I have repeatedly found that compassionately acknowledging the sensation of what *is* opens the door to what *could be.* Try it yourself and see.

CHAPTER 10

Upper and Mid Back: Thoracic Spine

Anatomy of the Thoracic Spine

The thoracic spine is composed of twelve vertebrae that ideally form a gentle posterior curve. The thoracic spine is designed mainly for rotational movement, lateral (side) bending, and forward bending (flexion), yet it also allows some extension (arching). Each vertebra has a pair of ribs attached, one on each side. The ribs reach out and curve around to the front, creating a strong cage to protect the heart and lungs (Figure 10.1).

When the thoracic curve flattens or curves too much, the natural shock-absorber effect of a balanced spine is lost. The back can seem like an inflexible rod. Tight, tense muscles can add to the sense of rigidity and contribute to neck, shoulder, arm, and hand pain. Maintaining suppleness in the thoracic region enhances the health of our heart and reflects our emotional flexibility and responsiveness.

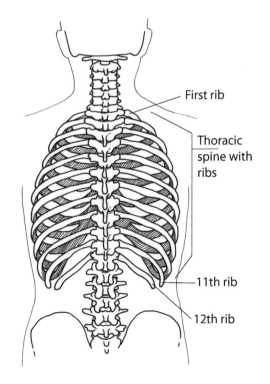

Fig. 10.1. Upper back with ribs, posterior view

First rib

Thoracic spine with ribs

11th rib

12th rib

Exercises to Enhance Flexibility in the Upper Back and Increase the Thoracic Curve

STERNUM FLEX: AWARENESS EXERCISE FOR THE THORACIC CURVE ,,,,,,,,,,,

This exercise provides a gentle way to tap into our awareness of the natural posterior curve of the upper back (thoracic spine) and the heart and lung space between the front of the chest and the spine.

This exercise comes from a meditation class[1] that included *mindful* movement. To me, moving mindfully means that we bring our attention to the specifics of how we move, noting from where the movement initiates, staying present with our sensations throughout the move, and perhaps sensing the effect of the movement within us.

➤ Sitting, lightly rest your fingers on your breastbone (sternum). Focus your attention on the contact point where your fingers meet the sternum. Allow movement to initiate from this contact by softly pushing with the fingers on the sternum, moving it slowly back toward the spine. Sense the thoracic spine naturally curling posterior in response. Allow your head to move from the spine in response—that is, don't initiate movement by moving your head forward. Keep your focus at the contact between the fingers and the sternum and monitor the movement from that interface (Figure 10.2).

When you have reached the furthest place of posterior curve, allow the sternum to initiate a forward (anterior) push toward the fingers. Notice the effect on your upper spine. Does it follow the breastbone or is it able to maintain some of its posterior curve while the sternum moves forward?

Gently and slowly repeat these movements. Sense the degree of flexibility in the thoracic area.

Next, you may want to include some of the variations:

- Push from the top, bottom, and middle of the sternum and notice the different sensations in your upper back.

- Take a deep breath as you push the sternum back. Does the breath support the movement of the upper spine?

- Try inhaling as you push from the sternum toward your fingers. Does the spine get drawn forward as if connected to the breastbone?

Notice the degree of flexibility in the area. Is it difficult to stick with the place of initiation or is there a tendency to initiate the movement from another area? It is easy to slip back into a familiar pattern of movement and initiate this from your lower ribs, your shoulders, or from your neck.

Take care to keep your attention at your sternum and initiate from the finger contact there while noting the effect in your upper back.

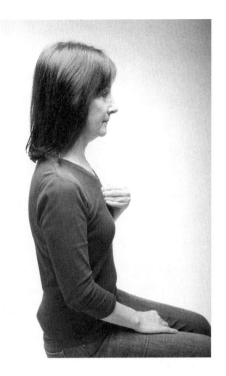

Fig. 10.2. Sternum flex

DISC FLUFFER: MOVEMENT EXERCISE TO REEDUCATE THE THORACIC CURVE (FOR THE UPPER BACK)

The gentle bouncing in this and the following exercise helps to warm and soften the gelatinous discs between each vertebra and reminds the spine of its potential for a relaxed thoracic curve. Once again, bringing awareness to the sensations in the upper back as you do this exercise increases its effectiveness.

➤ Sit in a chair, with your arms crossed over your chest, and allow your head to roll forward, bringing your spine into a natural backward (posterior) curl. Sense the subtle changes in the thoracic (upper back) area as the weight of your head drops forward toward your chest. Notice any tension or pulling between your shoulder blades, at the base of your neck, or in your lower back.

Staying curled, bring your attention to your upper back, and from there gently begin a gentle bouncing movement in your upper spine. See if you can sense the bouncing movement at each vertebra.

As you bounce, your head will slowly move toward your lap, but you are not initiating the movement from your neck or head but rather at the spine itself. As you continue to bounce, allow your body to roll forward and your upper back to curl even more.

When you have reached a comfortable forward limit, sense the curl of the thoracic area, and then while continuing the gentle bounce, begin to uncurl the spine, bouncing at each vertebra level as you rise from the lower vertebrae back to an upright posture (Figures 10.3 to 10.9).

Practice this exercise once or twice daily as a way to "fluff" your discs and reinstate a healthy thoracic curve.

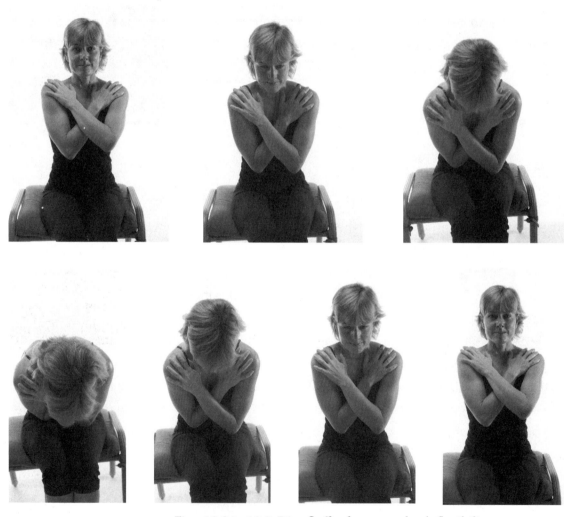

Figs. 10.3 to 10.9. Disc fluffer for upper-back flexibility

ROTATING DISC FLUFFER

In this variation of the above exercise you rotate (twist) the spine before beginning the gentle bouncing movement that softly "fluffs" the gelatinous discs that serve as shock absorbers for your spine.

➤ As above, sit with arms crossed over your chest, holding onto the opposite shoulder. Allow your head to roll slightly forward, bringing the spine into a natural posterior curl. Then rotate (twist) to one side and begin the gentle bouncing movement in your upper spine and allow your body to roll further into a curled position. When you have reached a comfortable forward limit, slowly begin to uncurl the spine, bouncing at each vertebra level as you gradually rise to an upright posture (Figures 10.10 to 10.13).

Rotate your spine to the opposite side and repeat the gentle bouncing on this side as well (Figures 10.14 to 10.17).

Do these movement exercises just once daily for two to three months to reestablish and rebalance the thoracic curve.

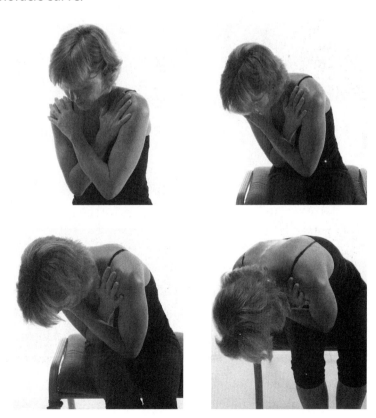

Figs. 10.10 to 10.13.
Rotating Disc Fluffer

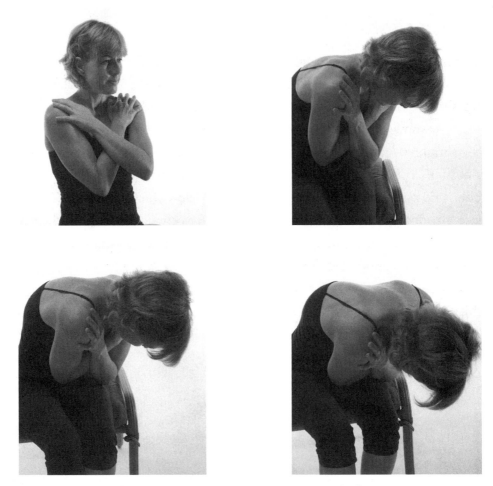

Figs. 10.14 to 10.17. Rotating Disc Fluffer

AWARENESS AND VISUALIZATION EXERCISE
FOR OPENING THE CHEST AND THORACIC AREA //

I remember my astonishment when I discovered how directly imagination can affect my physical comfort.

Here is an exercise from Gerda Alexander[2] that illustrates the importance of attention, visualization, and surrender in the process of self-care.

The purpose of the first part of the exercise is to take note of any restrictions, tension, holding, or resistance. Just breathe and notice where your body moves comfortably and where you feel tightness or strain. Bring your attention to the rib cage, the diaphragm, the muscles of the upper chest, shoulder, and arm. Notice where there is ease and which areas feel tight.

➤ Lying on your side, straighten the bottom leg and bend your top knee, rolling your top knee forward to rest on the floor. You may place your bottom hand on your knee if you like. Slowly and gently allow your top shoulder to rotate back toward the floor (away from your knee).

Notice your breath. Notice how far you can easily and comfortably move your shoulder while continuing to rest your top knee on the floor. As you breathe, notice any restrictions or areas of holding in the spine, ribs, shoulder, lower back, or pelvis. Notice any resistance to movement or to the breath. Just notice—don't try to push through any resistance. Stay within your range of comfort (Figure 10.18).

After a minute or so of just breathing and noticing in this position, slowly roll back into a resting position lying on your back.

Take your focus inside. Visualize the space between your spine and sternum and slowly move your awareness from the middle of your body out toward the shoulder, though the armpit, and into the arm of the side that you just stretched. Explore the inner territory of your upper torso with your mind's eye. You may notice the bones of the spine, the sternum, the ribs; or the muscles and tissues connecting one part to another; or the heart and lung. Imagine the fluids moving through the area. Quietly and calmly navigate from the sternum out to the arm, imagining or sensing the quality of the space, the tissue, the muscles, and the bones (Figure 10.19).

After two or three minutes in this relaxation and visualization, slowly return to the side-lying position with the top knee bent and the shoulder rotated back (Figure 10.20). Note any differences in your range of the movement or in the quality of the tissue, the muscles, the bones, or the skin. Is there an increase in your comfort level? Do the areas where you noticed holding or restriction feel more open or relaxed?

Repeat the exercise on the other side.

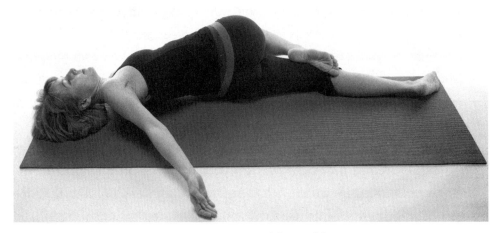

Fig. 10.18. Rotated "stretch"

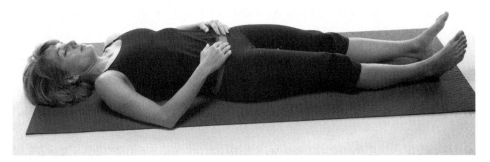

Fig. 10.19. Visualization exercise

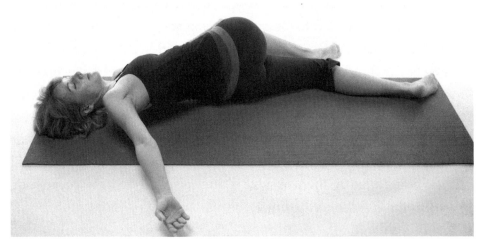

Fig. 10.20. Repeat rotated "stretch"

AWARENESS EXERCISE: FINDING THE THORACIC FLEXION REFLEX „„„„„„„„„

In one particular class I took with Gerda Alexander[2] she asked us to lie quietly on our back on the floor. We were to focus on one of our thoracic vertebrae, and to slowly move that one vertebra back toward the floor. As a group of respectful students we all did our best, but the frustration in the room was obvious. Gerda walked around and noted all means of trying going on. "We are not using our tongues this time," she would say. "Just the vertebra is moving." It seemed she was asking us to do the impossible. Finally, she decided that we needed a clue. The clue came in the form of this exercise.

This subtle movement exercise attunes our awareness to the reflexive activity stimulated in the upper back as we walk and also clarifies the direct relationship between walking and the health and flexibility of the thoracic spine.

➤ Lie on your back perpendicular to a nearby wall with your knees bent. Raise your lower legs and place your feet against the wall, creating a right angle between the wall and your lower legs. Your feet, knees, and hips should be aligned, with your lower legs parallel to floor, and the upper legs (hips to knees) parallel to the wall. It is important to maintain your lumbar curve while you do this exercise (you may use a rolled towel placed behind your waist).

Gently press your feet into the wall. Sense the reflexive movement in your upper back as your thoracic vertebrae curve (flex) slightly toward the floor (Figure 10.21).

If you are not sensing this subtle movement, you may need to fine-tune your initial set-up. Try placing your buttocks closer to the wall, but remember to keep your lower legs (knees to feet) parallel to the floor.

Experiment with this a bit: Instead of pushing into both legs, press one foot into the wall at a time.

Having fractured my thoracic spine in three places, I noted that the reflexes on one side of my spine worked well when I pressed either the right or left foot, but I could not sense any reflex activity on the other side of my spine. My accident had upset the reflexes in that area. Gerda assured me that my reflexes would return if I practiced this exercise. They have.

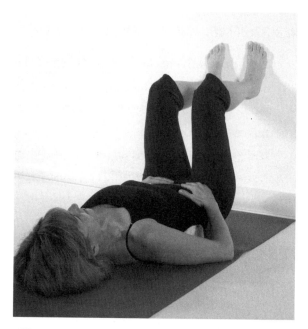

Fig. 10.21. Upper back (thoracic) flexion reflex

RELEASE POSITION FOR THORACIC ROTATION PREFERENCE ,,,,,,,,,,,,,,,,,,,,,,,,,,,,

When our reflexes are tuned, we balance quickly. Notice how easily we can increase our comfortable range of motion by acknowledging and affirming our preferences.

➤ Sitting, cross your arms and place your hands on your shoulders. Gently rotate your spine to the right. Stop rotating and allow your spine to bounce (rebound) back to midline. Then rotate your spine to the left and allow it to rebound back to center (Figures 10.22 to 10.24).

In which direction do you turn most easily? Notice the quality and tone within the rebound. Rotate to the most comfortable direction and stay there about twenty seconds, then slowly return to midline. Then check for increased range of motion and comfort or a more balanced tone in the opposite direction.

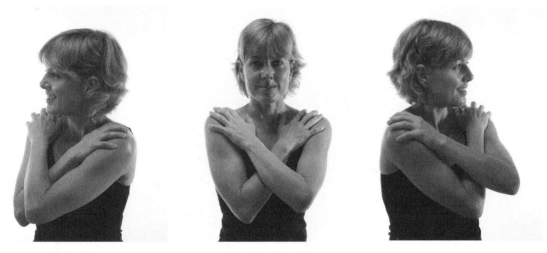

Figs. 10.22 to 10.24. Check for rotation preference

RELEASE POSITION FOR LATERAL-BEND PREFERENCE

Now check for lateral (side) bending preference.

➤ Sitting, side-bend to the right, bringing your right shoulder toward your right hip. Be careful to keep your head, neck, and upper body in the same plane as the hips, as if between two panes of glass. Note any tension, restriction, or pain as you make the movement. Return to center (Figures 10.25 and 10.26).

Next, laterally bend to the left, bringing your left shoulder toward the left hip with the same considerations (Figure 10.27). In which direction do you experience greater ease and comfort?

Repeat the side bend toward the comfortable direction and hold that position for ten to thirty seconds. Then recheck for increased range of motion or comfort in the opposite direction.

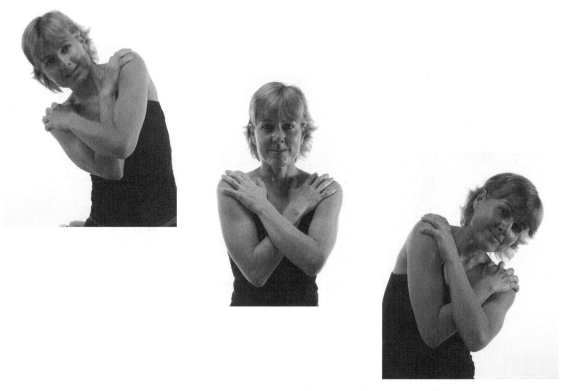

Figs. 10.25 to 10.27. Check side bending preference

COMBINING ROTATION AND LATERAL-BEND PREFERENCES,,,,,,,,,,,,,,,,,,,,,,,,,,,,,,,,,,

This exercise of combining the two preferences is good for rib pain as well as the tension of scoliosis. (See also Chapter 19, "Scoliosis.")

➤ If you feel pain or restriction on one side in the rib cage, try combining your lateral-bend preference with your rotation preference, so you'll be combining the pain-free movements. If you preferred rotating to the right and side-bending to the left, then slowly rotate to the right until you find your place of comfort and add a slight side bend to the left.

"Slow" is the key word here—move very slowly so you can sense the exact position where the tension releases and the pain disappears. Relax in this position for a minute or two and breathe, directing your exhalation to the area of holding (Figure 10.28).

Remember to come out of the position slowly so as not to reactivate the old holding pattern.

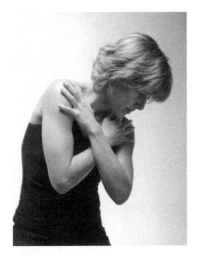

Fig. 10.28. Combining (left) rotation preference
with (left) side-bend preference

RELEASE POSITION FOR THE THORACIC AREA ///

➤ To release tension in the upper back, lie on your side with your knees bent and a pillow under your head. Your head, hips, and feet should be in a straight line. Bend your top elbow so your hand rests on your upper thigh. Slowly and gently let your top shoulder and elbow drop back toward the floor, resting where you have found the position of maximum relaxation (Figure 10.29).

Relax your whole body into this comfortable position. If it increases your comfort, place a pillow behind you as support for your arm (Figure 10.30).

Sleeping in this position can help to relieve hand and arm pain (see Chapter 14) and carpal tunnel symptoms. (For Carpal Tunnel Syndrome, see Chapter 20.) This position can also be combined with the Lazy Dog exercise in Chapter 3.

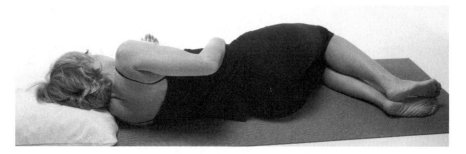

Fig. 10.29. Thoracic release position

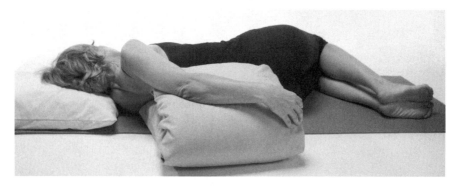

Fig. 10.30. Thoracic release with pillow

%% %% %%

The 12th Thoracic: A Transition Point in the Direction of the Natural Curves

The 12th thoracic vertebra is the lowest vertebra that has ribs attached—ribs that are very short and do not even reach as far as your sides. This area is vulnerable to strain and tension build-up for a number of reasons.

A balanced spine's natural curves create flexibility and shock absorption. However, inflexible postural patterns can cause strain and tension to develop at transition areas between the natural curves. At the 12th thoracic area, the posterior thoracic curve meets the anterior lumbar curve below it, and if the natural curves are not balanced, tightness and tension can develop. This same vulnerability manifests where the 5th lumbar (low back vertebra) meets the sacrum, and where the 7th cervical (neck vertebra) meets the 1st thoracic (rib vertebra).

Tension around the 12th thoracic can also come from a tight diaphragm muscle or a tense and contracted quadratus lumborum muscle (see Chapter 3).

Check the indicator point on the outside (lateral) upper edge of the hip bone. Tenderness here reflects tension at the 12th thoracic (Figure 10.31).

12TH THORACIC RELEASE: "ROAST TURKEY" ⁗⁗⁗⁗⁗⁗⁗⁗⁗⁗⁗⁗⁗⁗⁗⁗⁗⁗⁗⁗

This 12th Thoracic Release, also known as the "Roast Turkey," is a key release for opening movement between the upper and lower back, and helping to free the movement of lymph fluid from the lower trunk and extremities. This simple position also helps to release tension in the diaphragm, the 12th rib, and upper psoas contractions. Use this if the indicator point at the lateral upper edge of the hip bone is tender or if there is tension in your diaphragm, under your rib cage, or behind your waist.

➤ Lie on your back and bend your knees, feet resting on the floor. Push into your feet so your buttocks lift up off the floor, and slip a pillow under your buttocks. For best results, keep the pillow below your waist.

Once in position, curl up by bringing your knees toward your shoulders. Let your knees fall open and out to the sides. Rest your elbows on the floor, so your hands reach up and support your knees (Figure 10.32). Allowing the elbows to rest on the floor keeps the arms relaxed. This position gets its nickname because your body is in a pose resembling that of a roast turkey on a platter!

Breathe slowly and evenly, allowing your diaphragm to expand in all directions. Let your exhalation be relaxed and slow. Try not to push or blow the breath out. Relax your mouth in a slightly open position and allow a slow, natural exhalation.

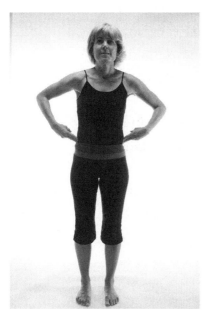

Fig. 10.31. 12th thoracic indicator points

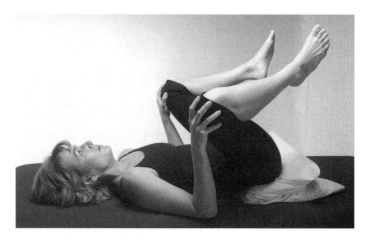

Fig. 10.32. "Roast Turkey" release for 12th thoracic

※ ※ ※

CHAPTER 11

Spinal Integrity

The Natural Curves of the Spine

Arthur Pauls, the founder of Ortho-Bionomy, would often lecture about the importance of balanced spinal curves. He once said, "There is not one country in the world that recognizes that your structure is important. No system works to balance the three spinal curves. The lumbar curve should be in the lumbar area, but in most people the lumbar curve extends up into the thoracic area."

He believed that a balanced thoracic curve is key to good posture and to an avoidance of heart problems in later life. A reversed thoracic curve—one in which the upper spine is dished inward—puts pressure on the heart because it limits the space in the upper chest. He spoke of an American doctor he met who said that every patient he saw with mitral valve[1] trouble had a flat thoracic spine.

Arthur noted:

In school you are taught to pull your shoulders back and stick your chest out. Sit up straight. That just creates a straight spine. A straight spine has no give. Yet every anatomy book in the world shows the three curves. Three curves give the spine flexibility and strength. Just like a suspension bridge has more flexibility and strength. If children were taught in school how to release and balance their curves, you wouldn't see so many back problems in later life.… [Ortho-Bionomy] is one of the only techniques that teaches you how to get your three curves back [into alignment].… If you take a spine that is curved and straighten it, it lengthens. How will that straight spine now fit in the body? It has to curve sideways, and then you develop scoliosis.

When the three curves of the spine are balanced, the whole body functions better.[2]

The places where the spinal curves change direction are the most natural places for tension to build up. For example, when someone has a flat thoracic curve or is lacking a proper lumbar curve, tension will build at the 7th cervical and 1st thoracic area, pushing the bones posterior and forming what is commonly called "dowager's hump."

Healthy Posture

Anatomy

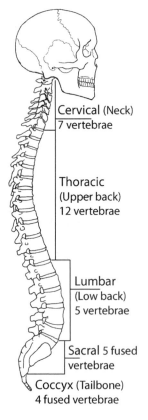

Cervical (Neck)
7 vertebrae

Thoracic
(Upper back)
12 vertebrae

Lumbar
(Low back)
5 vertebrae

Sacral 5 fused
vertebrae

Coccyx (Tailbone)
4 fused vertebrae

Vertebral Column
Right Lateral View

Healthy posture begins with balanced spinal structure. The five thick lumbar vertebrae of the lower back are designed to form a gentle forward (anterior) curve. The twelve vertebrae of the thoracic region (upper and mid back) form a backward (posterior) curve. The seven smaller cervical (neck) vertebrae gently curve anterior. In between and connecting each of the bony vertebrae are gelatinous discs that give our spine flexibility and support during movement. The discs and the spinal curves act as natural shock absorbers for the spine (Figure 11.1).

Fig. 11.1. Balanced spinal curves, side view. Courtesy of *Illustrated Essentials of Musculoskeletal Anatomy,* 4th Edition, by Sieg and Adams (Gainesville, FL: Megabooks, Inc., 1992); www.muscleanatomybook.com.

SUPPORTING THE NATURAL SPINAL CURVES WHILE YOU SLEEP,,,,,,,,,,,,,,,,,,,,,,

This exercise helps to reestablish our natural curves, allowing the spine to maintain its strength and flexibility.

➤ Fold two hand towels in half from top to bottom. Then fold the sides into the center and roll each towel into a cylinder (Figures 11.2 to 11.6). Place on the bed for use after the movement exercise. You may want to experiment with the thickness of the towels to determine what works best for you. You want the rolled towel to feel supportive under your neck and behind your waist. If it is too bulky, there may be too much pressure to those areas.

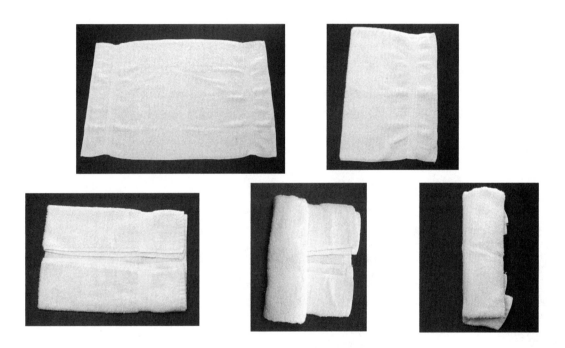

Figs. 11.2 to 11.6. Towel folds and roll

➤ Begin standing and lift your elbows to shoulder height with your fingertips overlapping at midline. Gently rotate the spine as far as is comfortable left and right. Let your eyes follow your elbows so your head rotates with the spine. Do this movement thirty to forty times in each direction (Figures 11.7 to 11.10). Rotating the spine warms and softens the gelatinous discs between the vertebrae.

Then lie down, placing one of the rolled towels under your waist and the other under your neck. Lie on your back with the rolled towels in position for at least twenty minutes (Figure 11.11). Once the discs are warmed, lying on the towels helps to reestablish the normal spinal curves. If comfortable, you may sleep in this position with the towels supporting the lumbar and cervical curves.

For a while, I was using only the neck roll. This didn't work as well, though, and I realized that giving support to both curves allowed my neck more relaxation and support. If you sleep with towel rolls, you may find that placing a pillow under your knees offers further support for your low back.

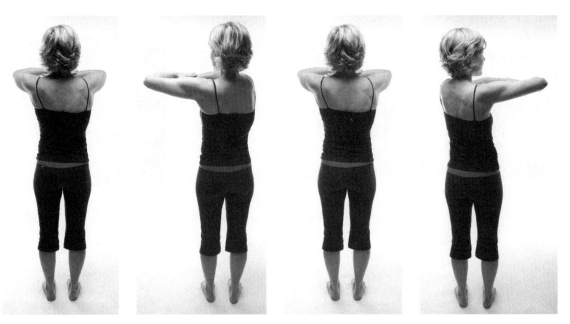

Figs. 11.7 to 11.10. Spinal rotation to warm discs

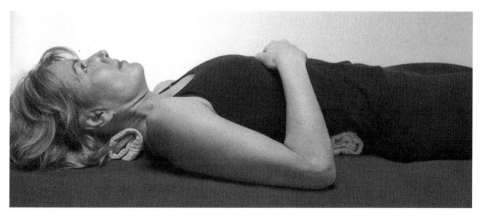

Fig. 11.11. Lie on rolled towels to reeducate spinal curves

⁂

More about Posture

Posture is the shape of our experience. Within our posture we can see our history. We are born with genetically inherited patterns of bone structure and body type. As children, we model our posture or manner of walking after our parents. Patterns of movement behavior are tacitly absorbed and normalized as our own. Falls, injuries, or emotional threats can create protective behaviors that leave traces of defensive patterning in the underlying structure.

Within posture we can also see our present. Our choice of activities and sports may determine if we become right- or left-side dominant. We may develop habitual patterns of use from the way we carry a baby on our hip, hold the phone to our ear while we type, or shoulder our computer as we travel. Our jobs, the way we drive, or even the habitual way we sit watching TV can create subtle imbalances over time. These patterns are visible in the wear pattern on our shoes, a favorite chair, and the seat of the car. We may also see evidence of them by looking objectively at our posture in the mirror.

There is some benefit to using the relative objectivity of observation. After my motorcycle accident my side-leaning posture caused the doctor to suggest that I practice standing and walking in front of a mirror. The side bend might have felt fine to me, but the longer I stayed in that habit, the more I was creating a sense of normalcy with it. I was also limiting my potential range of motion, and my body was forgetting that it had options for a more balanced posture.

Using the mirror to find good posture can be tricky, though, since what "looks right" can override your internal sense of alignment, balance, and comfort. In cases of injury or compensation, adding one holding pattern of "looks right" on top of another can create more tension. The solution here is not to move from a static side-leaning posture to a static upright posture and then try to hold the correct posture.

Posture is a dynamic balancing process between structure and function. By opening up our options through movement, and releasing the underlying tension and holding patterns through positioning, the body incorporates changes in an optimum and functional way. Reeducating the body through specific exercises of movement and positioning increases our sensory orientation capacity to naturally move toward balance. Gradually and gently, rigid patterns can be replaced with postural and functional ease.

Working with the following postural exercises daily over a period of three to six months will assist you in building healthier posture. These movement exercises specifically deal with balancing the spinal curves. Please also refer to the chapters on the low back (Chapter 2), the upper back (Chapter 10), and the neck (Chapter 15) for additional exercises and release positions for these areas of the spine. If you have scoliosis, please refer to Chapter 19.

Pelvis and Spine: The Foundation of Posture

Anatomy of the Pelvis

Although these areas are addressed individually earlier in the book, in this section on posture we work with the pelvis as a whole unit made up of parts.

The pelvis—or pelvic bowl, as it is sometimes called—is formed by the two hip bones, the sacrum, and the coccyx (tailbone). Each hip bone is actually formed by the fusion of three bones: the ilium (hip bone), the ischium (sit bone), and the pubis (pubic bone). Yet for the most part each side tends to move as one bone. Muscles, ligaments, and tendons connect all the bones and stabilize the pelvis for weight-bearing, weight-transference, and movement, while also serving as a supporting vessel for our pelvic organs (Figure 11.12).

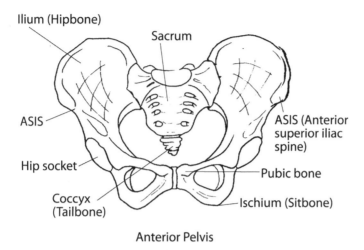

Fig. 11.12. Anterior female pelvis.
Extract from *Anatomy of Movement,* courtesy
of Blandine Calais Germain and Désiris Publishing, France.

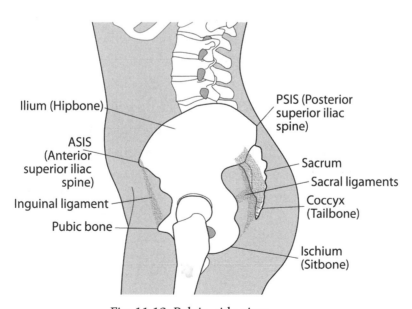

Fig. 11.13. Pelvis, side view

Reestablishing the Lumbar Curve

As we walk, the natural movement of the pelvis extends and flexes the lumbar curve. Often, low-back pain is caused by patterns of holding that immobilize the lumbar vertebrae.

This group of exercises uses movement to remind the neuromuscular system to recognize its options. They also aid in bringing balanced movement to the lumbar spine.

AWARENESS EXERCISE FOR SIT BONES ⁄⁄

I remember the first time my attention was drawn to my sit bones and to their contact with my chair. I began to slowly and subtly rock my hip bones forward and back, noticing the contact on my sit bones change and feeling the movement in my spine. If I did the movement very slowly, I could sense the way I was using my hip muscles on both sides, and I became aware of subtle imbalances from one side to the other. I continued to practice this movement and to note an increased comfort and relaxation in my lower back.

Arthur Pauls had taught that this relaxed forward-and-back pelvic movement would help to reeducate the natural spinal curves and bring increased flexibility to the spine. Imagine my delight during the next posture class with Arthur when he found that my scoliosis had corrected.

➤ While sitting in a chair, notice how you are sitting on your sit bones. Without shifting, feel your weight on them. Do you feel more weight on one side than the other? Don't try to correct it—just notice. If it helps, you can slide your hands under your buttocks and feel with your hands how your weight is distributed in each of the sit bones (Figures 11.14 and 11.15).

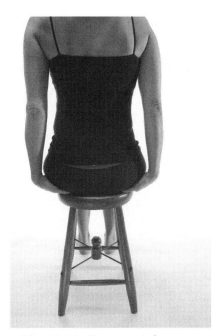

Fig. 11.14. Contact sit bones

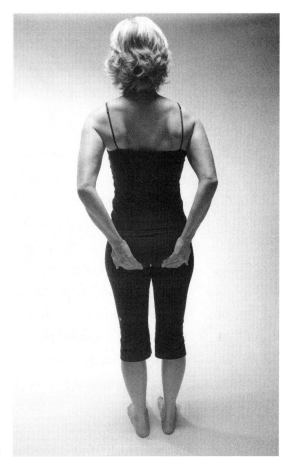

Fig. 11.15. Locate sit bones

FINDING THE MIDPOINT OF PELVIC ROTATION

This exercise introduces balanced movement to your lower back. Rather than imposing a new postural holding pattern, we offer the body movement options and allow the self-balancing reflexes to work from within. In this way, we come to a natural balance within the spine, rather than creating new tension patterns by trying to hold a posture.

This exercise can be done frequently during the day, especially if you have a job that requires sitting. The exercise can be very restful to the lumbar (lower) back and will allow the natural curves to strengthen and support the spine. Just remember to stay in your comfort zone here and not move any further than is comfortable.

➤ Place your hands on top of your hip bones and imagine that they are tricycle wheels. Rotate the wheels (of the pelvis) forward as far as is comfortable, so you create an anterior (forward) curve in your lower back (Figure 11.16).

Then rock back as far as is comfortable until your lower back is flat or has a slight posterior (backward) curve. Initiate this movement at the sacral and lumbar area of the pelvis or even from your sit bones, not at the waist, chest, shoulders, or head. Placing your hands on your hips helps to focus and initiate the movement from the pelvis. Do this movement slowly without moving your upper body forward (Figure 11.17).

Allow the movement in your lower back to come from the forward/back rotation of the hips. As you move, notice if there are any places that hesitate or jerk, and notice where the range of movement seems smooth. Try to move slowly enough that the muscles on both sides begin to work together for smooth, coherent movement. Rotate the pelvis forward and back four or five times, moving as far as you comfortably can.

Now, shorten the range a little bit at each end, i.e., move forward but not quite as far, and then move back but not quite as far. Continue shortening the range a little with each forward and backward movement until the midpoint is reached. At the midpoint, tune into your sit bones and the lower back (Figure 11.18). Do you sense relaxation in your spine? Do you feel the support of the pelvis under your torso?

Once you have found the midpoint and allowed yourself to sense the ease in the spine and the foundation of support in the sit bones and the pelvic floor, return to your normal daily activities. Don't try to hold this posture. The body is smart and will integrate the changes that are introduced at a pace that can be structurally supported.

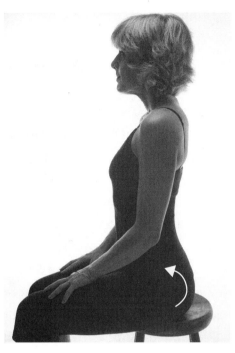

Fig. 11.16. Rotate pelvis forward

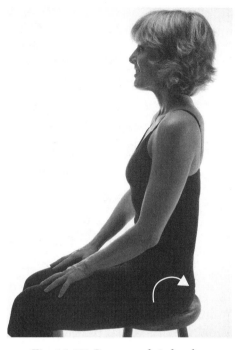

Fig. 11.17. Rotate pelvis back

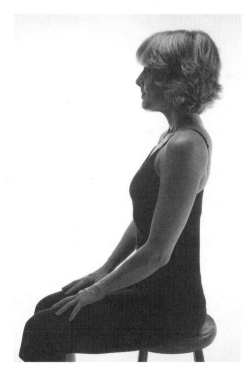

Fig. 11.18. Midpoint

DISC FLUFFER TO REESTABLISH THE THORACIC CURVE,,

The next exercise was first introduced in Chapter 10. It is repeated here for its role in spinal posture.

The gentle bouncing in this and the following exercise helps to warm and soften the gelatinous discs between each vertebra and reminds the spine of its potential for a relaxed thoracic curve. Once again, bringing awareness to the sensations in the upper back as you do this exercise increases its effectiveness.

➤ Sitting in a chair, with your arms crossed over your chest, allow your head to roll forward, bringing your spine into a natural backward (posterior) curl (Figure 11.19). Sense the subtle changes in the thoracic area as the weight of your head slowly drops forward toward your chest. Notice any tension or pulling between your shoulder blades, at the base of your neck, or in your lower back.

Staying curled, bring your attention to your upper back, and from there gently begin a gentle bouncing movement in your upper spine. See if you can sense the bouncing movement at each vertebra level. As you bounce, your head will slowly move toward your lap, but you are not initiating the movement from your neck or head but rather at the spine itself. As you continue to bounce, allow your body to roll forward and your upper back to curl even more. When you have reached a comfortable forward limit, sense the curl of the thoracic area and then, while continuing the gentle bounce, begin to uncurl the spine, bouncing at each vertebra level as you rise from the lower vertebrae back to an upright posture. Practice this exercise once or twice daily as a way to "fluff" your discs and reinstate a healthy thoracic curve (Figures 11.20 to 11.23).

To further increase mobility in the upper spine, also use the "Sternum Flex" and other exercises in Chapter 10.

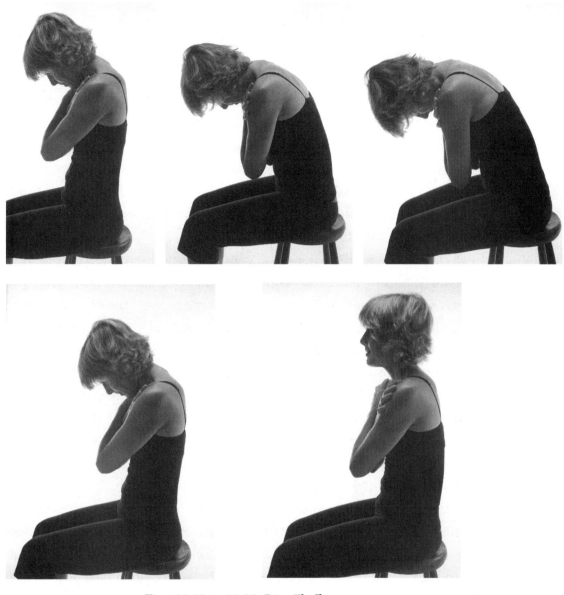

Figs. 11.19 to 11.23. Disc Fluffer
to enhance natural curve of the upper back

Balanced Sitting Posture

COMBINING DISC FLUFFER WITH FINDING YOUR MIDPOINT ,,,,,,,,,,,,,,,,,,,,,,,,,

When this exercise is done well, you will begin to reeducate the lumbar curve to the most functional midpoint, and the upper back to its more natural posterior curve. You should feel more relaxed in your shoulders and more balanced in your spine, with the weight supported by the pelvis.

➤ As in the basic Disc Fluffer exercise, cross your arms over your chest, roll your head forward, and begin a gentle bouncing movement as you allow your thoracic spine to curl forward (Figure 11.24).

Then, with your head down and your thoracic spine rounded, rotate your pelvis ("tricycle wheels") forward just to the midpoint that you located in "Finding the Midpoint of Pelvic Rotation," two exercises above in this chapter. Be sure you are initiating the movement in your pelvis and not from your waist or upper body (Figure 11.25).

Once you have arrived at your midpoint with your head down and chin tucked, maintain the curl in the upper spine while slowly allowing your curled upper spine to move directly back until your shoulders are directly aligned over your hips. At this point your chin is still tucked and the upper back maintains a slight posterior curve; your shoulders are aligned over your hips. Now slowly raise your head to upright (Figures 11.26 and 11.27).

Monitor yourself and your sensations carefully, so you don't simply resume your familiar pattern. The most common mistakes in this exercise are initiating movement to the midpoint from waist or rib level and pulling the shoulders back by straightening the spine and thereby losing the thoracic curve.

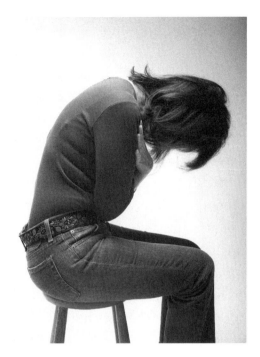

Fig. 11.24. Disc fluffer

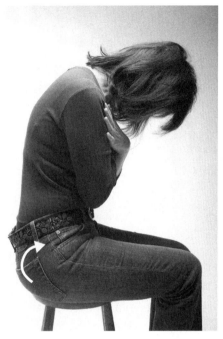

Fig. 11.25. Rotate hips to midpoint

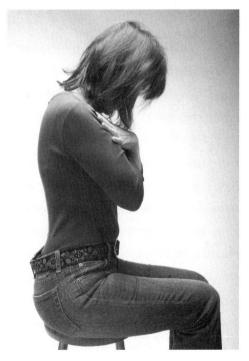

Fig. 11.26. Bring shoulders over hips

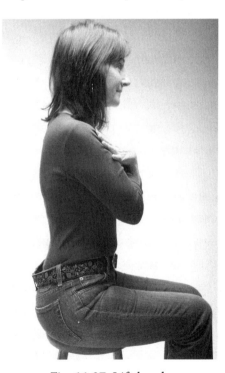

Fig. 11.27. Lift head

A Word about Sugar

Years after my motorcycle accident, I took a class in meditation. I noticed my body relaxing during the quiet sitting practice. As my shoulders dropped, I began to sense a burning, searing pain in my thoracic spine in the area of the "healed" compressed fractures. When I tensed my shoulders and lifted the weight up off my mid-spine, the pain disappeared.

This made me curious—my challenge became: Could I relax my shoulders and release the tension and pain in my spine at the same time? One day I noticed a Touch for Health Chart,[3] and my attention was drawn to the latissimus dorsi muscle, a large, wide muscle originating at the low back and lower ribs and extending up the back, across the lower part of the shoulder blade, then wrapping under the arm, where it attaches onto the top front of the arm. Since this area of my back often hurt and felt weak, and since it attached to the areas where my spine had been broken, I wondered if weakness in this muscle could be causing the pain I felt in my spine.

Touch for Health is a system that correlates information about acupuncture, muscle strength, and nutrition for the support of postural balance. The chart showed a relationship between the large latissimus dorsi muscle and the pancreas, suggesting that sweets in the diet could cause this muscle to weaken.

I began an experiment to see if eliminating sweets could help my back pain and allow my shoulders to relax. Over time, I found that avoiding sweets did calm the hyper reflexive muscle tension patterns in my back and shoulders that caused my mid-back pain. By strengthening the latissimus dorsi muscle with exercise and disciplining myself around sugar, I began to stabilize and maintain spinal strength and postural balance without tension and pain.

Often clients and students with instability or pain and tension in the thoracic spine respond positively when asked if they have been eating more sweets lately. The recognition of this potential relationship between sugar intake and back pain allows more control and choice about our comfort levels. This same thoracic area of the body can benefit from the 12th Thoracic Release or "Roast Turkey" exercise.

CHAPTER 12

Ribs

Anatomy of the Ribs

We have twenty-four ribs, composed of twelve pairs that connect to both sides of each thoracic vertebra. They form a protective cage for the soft organs, curving around from the spine and attaching in the front to the breastbone (sternum), either directly or by means of cartilage. The last two ribs—the 11th and 12th—are shorter and are known as "floating" ribs since they do not have a front (anterior) attachment (Figures 12.1 and 12.2). Muscles called intercostals attach to the top of one rib and the bottom of the next in a crosswise pattern, making the protective structure of the rib cage flexible.

Pain in the rib cage can result from falls, injuries, or strains that cause a torque or tension in the muscles between the ribs, or from tension and pulls in the large domed-shaped diaphragm muscle that extends beneath the bottom of the ribs to form the floor of the thoracic area.

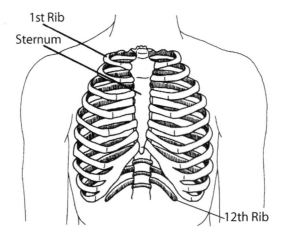

Fig. 12.1. Anterior rib cage

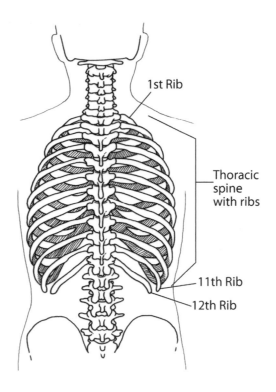

Fig. 12.2. Posterior rib cage

❦❦❦

General Release Positioning for the Rib Cage

➤ For tenderness on the side of the rib cage, slowly side-bend (shoulder to hip) and rotate the torso, curving around the tender point until tenderness is relieved (Figure 12.3).

Move slowly in an exploratory manner to locate the release position. Quicker movements tend to skip past the position of optimal relief.

If general positioning doesn't seem to work, try the more subtle releases for working with individual ribs presented below.

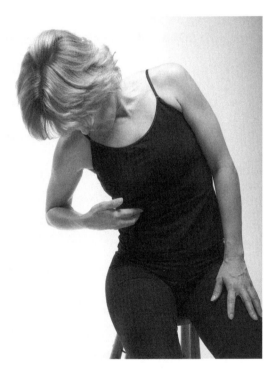

Fig. 12.3. Side-bend and curl around sore rib

DIAPHRAGM RELEASE //

The diaphragm, made up of muscle fibers arched in the shape of a dome, spans the bottom of the rib cage. The diaphragm has attachments to the bottom of the sternum, the inner side of the 10th, llth, and 12th ribs (lower six ribs), and the central tendon extending from the front of the 12th thoracic to the 2nd lumbar vertebra. The dome is arched in a relaxed position at exhalation and flattens at inhalation. Tensions or pulls in the diaphragm can create internal pressures against the rib cage (Figure 12.4).

This exercise can help to release diaphragm tension. Try also 12th Thoracic Release, "Roast Turkey" (Chapter 10), for releasing the diaphragm (Figure 12.5).

➤ In a sitting position, use your fingers to feel underneath the rib cage for tightness or muscular tension (Figure 12.6).

Slowly bend, using a combination of side bending and rotation to curve around the tight area, creating a "cave" around the tension. Move slowly so you can feel the position that creates maximum softening of the tissue (Figure 12.7).

Stay in this position for a minimum of twenty seconds, relaxing and gently breathing into the area.

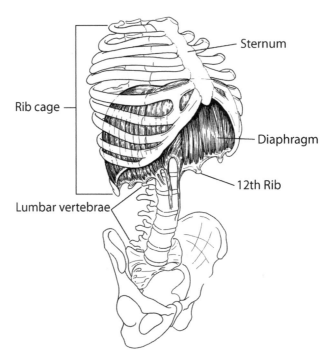

Fig. 12.4. Diaphragm. Courtesy of *Illustrated Essentials of Musculoskeletal Anatomy,* 4th Edition, by Sieg and Adams (Gainesville, FL: Megabooks, Inc., 1992), www.muscleanatomybook.com

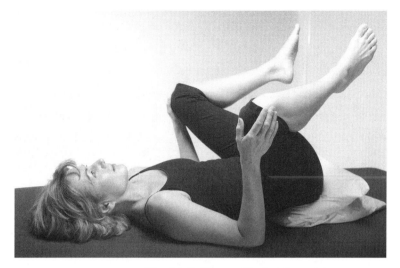

Fig. 12.5. "Roast Turkey" position

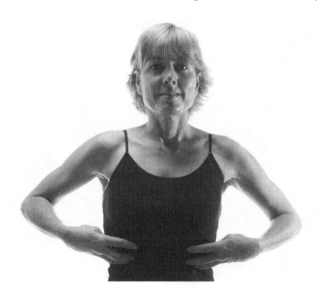

Fig. 12.6. Diaphragm points

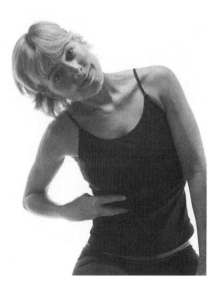

Fig. 12.7. Diaphragm release

❧❧❧

1st Rib (Top of Shoulder)

The isometric movement to release the 1st rib also helps to release shoulder and lower neck tension, and to open up the area for better lymph drainage. For any tension or discomfort in the shoulders, chest, neck, arms, and even the hands and fingers, release the 1st rib first.

The 1st rib curves upward from its attachment at the sternum, goes directly under the clavicle, and connects to the 1st thoracic vertebra in the back. A contraction of muscles around the 1st rib is often responsible for tension in the neck and top of the shoulder. Releasing it is essential preparation for other shoulder releases.

Tension in this area may block the flow of lymph fluid from the head and neck, resulting in greater congestion in the head, sinuses, and chest. These techniques, therefore, are also useful for treating the symptoms of a cold.

You can assess for tension at the 1st rib by feeling (palpating) for tension at the top of your shoulders just adjacent to the lower neck. If there is tension, release the 1st rib.

Two releases are presented. They may seem a bit complicated at first, but please persevere, for they can be very effective at relieving tension and discomfort in the shoulder region. Try them both to see which one works best for you.

ISOMETRIC RELEASE FOR THE 1ST RIB

➤ Sit on a chair and bend your knee, placing your foot on the edge of the chair. You may also do this exercise by standing or sitting, directly facing a table or shelf surface that is shoulder height. This surface or your knee will offer resistance for the isometric.

Bend your elbow and rest it on a sturdy surface or your bent knee. Initiate a small push (twenty percent or less of your strength) from the elbow into the knee or surface. Maintain this isometric pressure for ten seconds while visualizing the elbow pushing down through the surface (Figure 12.8).

After ten seconds of attempted movement, release the push and let the elbow drop to your side. Gently and slowly raise the elbow directly out to the side (perpendicular to the torso) and lean the elbow into the wall to bring compression to the shoulder joint. Allow the muscles in the neck and shoulder area to relax completely. Maintain this relaxed position for ten to thirty seconds (Figures 12.9 and 12.10).

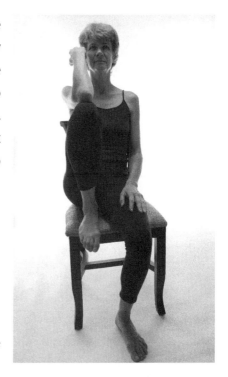

Fig. 12.8. Push elbow into knee

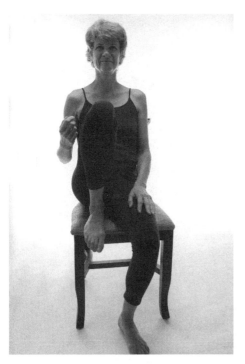

Fig. 12.9. Release elbow toward floor

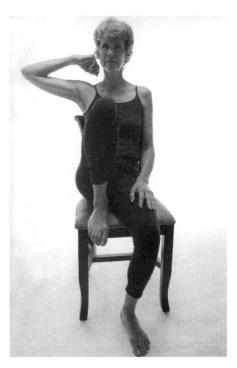

Fig. 12.10. Bring elbow perpendicular to body and lean into wall

ALTERNATIVE ISOMETRIC RELEASE FOR THE 1ST RIB ,,

➤ Place a soft pillow over the back of a kitchen or desk chair. Sitting sideways on the chair, hang the arm of the affected (painful, tight) side over the back of the chair so that your armpit rests on the pillow. Gently reach the hand of the affected side down toward the floor, using the rib muscles to assist in the reaching (Figure 12.11). The pillow on the chair back will provide soft resistance to the movement.

Continue the isometric pulling for ten seconds and then stand up, allowing the arm to passively drop toward the floor, completing the attempted movement (Figure 12.12).

Next, bend the elbow, raise your arm out to the side perpendicular to the torso and level with the shoulder, and lean your elbow into the wall, allowing the muscles in the neck and shoulder area to relax completely. Maintain this relaxed position for a minimum of ten to thirty seconds (Figure 12.13).

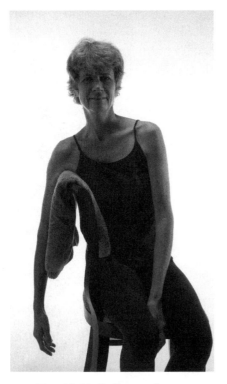

Fig. 12.11. Pull arm down

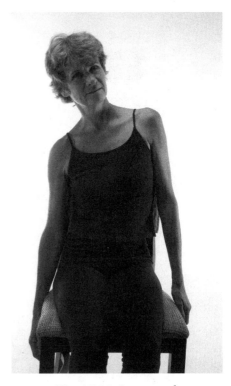

Fig. 12.12. Let arm drop

Fig. 12.13. Bring arm perpendicular to body and lean into wall

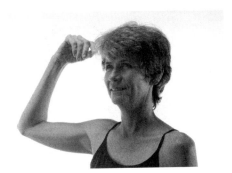

RIB RELEASE AT BREASTBONE POINTS ,,

Releasing tender points along the breastbone (sternum) frees the ribs and also helps to rebalance lymph flow and optimize health.[1]

➤ Check for tenderness along the edges of your breastbone where the ribs meet the sternum. If any areas are tender, gently bend forward and rotate slightly to create a "cave" around the point (Figures 12.14 and 12.15).

You may also gently grasp the upper arm on the same side and bring it over toward the tender point, curling your body around the point until you sense a softening there.

Relax in this positioning for at least ten to twenty seconds.

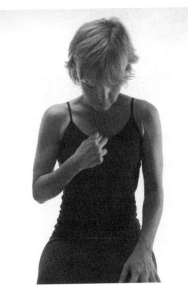

Fig. 12.14. Locate painful rib

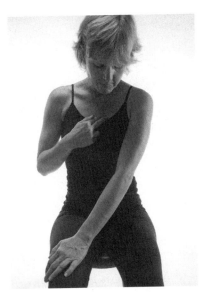

Fig. 12.15. Release position for rib pain near sternum

SUBTLE MOVEMENTS FOR RELEASING INDIVIDUAL RIB TENSION ˌˌˌˌˌˌˌˌˌˌˌˌˌ

Working with individual ribs can often bring a sense of essential relief at a more internal or emotional level. The intercostal muscles that lie between adjacent ribs need only a tiny bit of movement to release, so working with the individual ribs tends to be subtle. The trick is to find the preferred direction of movement and to touch the rib very softly, listening with the fingertips and internally for the slightest sense of ease.

➤ Sitting or lying in a comfortable position, use your middle finger to gently feel for tenderness, pain, or tension any place along a rib. With the fingertip lightly touching the skin, very gently explore movement preferences at the skin level by moving slowly in each of the various directions around the point of tenderness until you find a direction where the skin moves easily and tenderness disappears. Continue to hold the fingertip in this position for a minute or so (Figure 12.16).

Remember to breathe and relax the whole body while allowing the release to integrate.

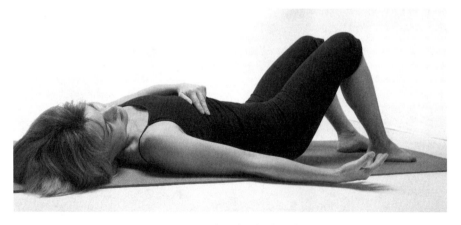

Fig. 12.16. Individual rib release

FIGURE-EIGHT MOVEMENT EXERCISE
TO MAINTAIN FLEXIBILITY IN THE RIBS ,,,

The object here is to open up movement in the rib cage by tracing a figure-eight pattern laterally (sideways) across the rib cage, exploring the range of motion available within the ribs.

➤ Standing, place your hands around the bottom of your rib cage with thumbs in front and fingers in back. Gently push your right hand into the posterior right ribs, moving them diagonally toward the left front. Then curve from the left front toward the left back in a circular way, exploring the potential within this range of motion. Now push with your left hand diagonally from the left back ribs to the right front, and then curve the right ribs in a circular way out to the side and toward the right back (Figures 12.17 to 12.20).

Move your hand position up along the sides of the rib cage and repeat the movement sequence from different starting points.

Reverse the direction by pushing with the left thumb diagonally to the right posterior and curve around on the right to the front; then from the right thumb push into the ribs, moving them diagonally toward the left back then once again curling around to the left front. Continue to repeat the sideways figure eights, exploring and opening the movement capacity of the rib cage.

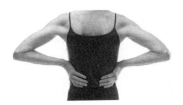

Fig. 12.17. Hands at lower ribs

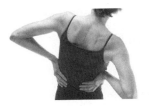

Fig. 12.18. Right hand pushes diagonally toward left front

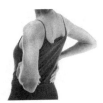

Fig. 12.19. Left elbow swings back

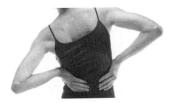

Fig. 12.20. Left hand pushes ribs diagonally toward right front

Figures 12.17 to 12.20. Figure-Eight movement for ribs

%%%

CHAPTER 13

Shoulders

The shoulders are frequently the place where we carry and experience tension. I often muse that "shoulder" is spelled like the word "should" with an "er" (emergency room) component. Are people with chronic shoulder complaints hounded by a sense of the "shoulds" in their lives? Is there an urgency to all these "shoulds" that increases the sense of pressure and tension? Metaphorically, we may have a multitude of plates spinning on sticks in the air, and it is the shoulders' job not to let any of the plates drop. All of the energy goes into the spinning rather than into the completion of the task at hand. Keeping those plates in the air can be exhausting, because the shoulders never get a chance to rest.

In my experience, chronic shoulder tension is best addressed as a full body response. When the spine is aligned and balanced, strong and flexible, the shoulders can rest down. The spine, in turn, depends on the low back and pelvis to serve as its foundation. All together, we're looking at postural balance to support the shoulders.

Keep in mind when working with shoulder tension:

- Exercises and releases for thoracic, lumbar, and cervical spine
- Releases for 1st and 3rd ribs and rib flexibility
- Postural exercises for pelvic rotation
- If hounded by projects that you think you "should" get done, prioritize, focus, finish one thing, and call that "complete" for the moment.

Anatomy of the Shoulder

The shoulder supports the arm's connection to the body and is responsible for movement of the arm. Three bones come together to form the shoulder joint: the collarbone (clavicle), shoulder blade (scapula), and upper arm bone (humerus). The clavicle attaches to the sternum and is the only bony connection that the shoulder girdle makes with the upright (axial) skeleton. A complex system of muscle groups attaches the arm to the torso and supports the movement of the arm in the joint (Figures 13.1 to 13.3).

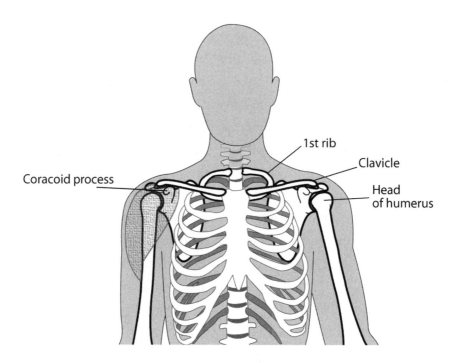

Fig. 13.1. Anterior shoulder

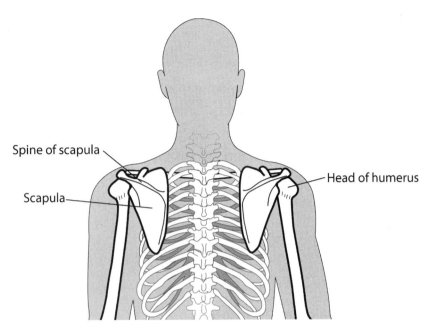

Fig. 13.2. Posterior shoulder

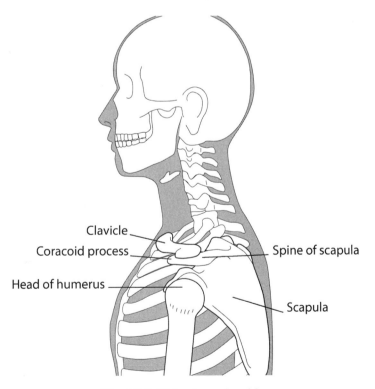

Fig. 13.3. Side view, shoulder

General Release Movements for the Shoulder

Many of these exercises are designed to release the shoulders by initiating movement from the hand or arm to allow the shoulder to move more passively. Moving from the farther end (peripheral or distal end) breaks up our common tendency to initiate all movement from the same place, which leads to overuse. When the muscles learn to organize differently for movement, new options arise, and tense and painful patterns are interrupted.

SWIMMING RECEPTIONIST

This is an excellent exercise for those who sit at a computer or answer phones. The movement is initiated in the hands, allowing the shoulders to move more passively. Do this one a few times throughout the day to relax shoulder tension.

➤ Standing, extend your arms out in front of your chest with the palms turned up. Slowly turn the palms of your hands toward your face, and then slowly bring your hands to your face. As your hands near the face, turn the palms inward and down and then continue the movement forward again to full extension of the arms. Then turn your palms up again and repeat the sequence, keeping the movement fluid as if swimming (Figures 13.4 to 13.10).

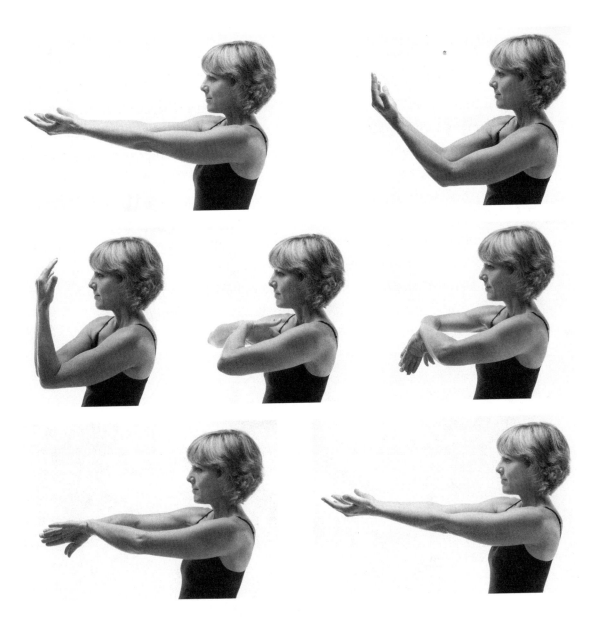

Figs. 13.4 to 13.10. Swimming Receptionist

FLOURISHES,,,

➤ Standing with your arms resting at your side, initiate tiny flourishing movements from your fingers as if you were turning a coin between them. Increase the finger movements to begin including your hand and wrist. Notice as you make the movements a bit larger how your lower arm and elbow become involved.

Allow the movement to influence your upper arm and shoulder, eventually moving in larger and larger flourishing patterns. Remember to check in and be sure that the fingers are initiating the movement, with the arm and shoulder merely following (Figures 13.11 to 13.16).

Initiating movement from the periphery allows the core patterns in the arm and shoulder to rest and learn new pain-free options.

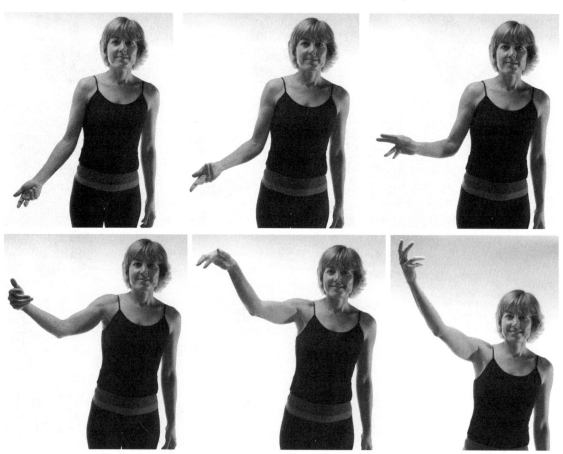

Figs. 13.11 to 13.16. Flourishes

DOORKNOBS ///

➤ Stand with your arms at your side, and imagine that you have doorknobs in your hands. Begin rotation movements in the wrists as if turning the door-knobs, first in one direction and then the other. Notice how the rotational movement in the wrist causes the lower arm to rotate, and the elbow and shoulder to rotate as well.

Slowly, while continuing to turn the doorknobs, raise hands and arms sideways away from the body (Figures 13.17 to 13.22).

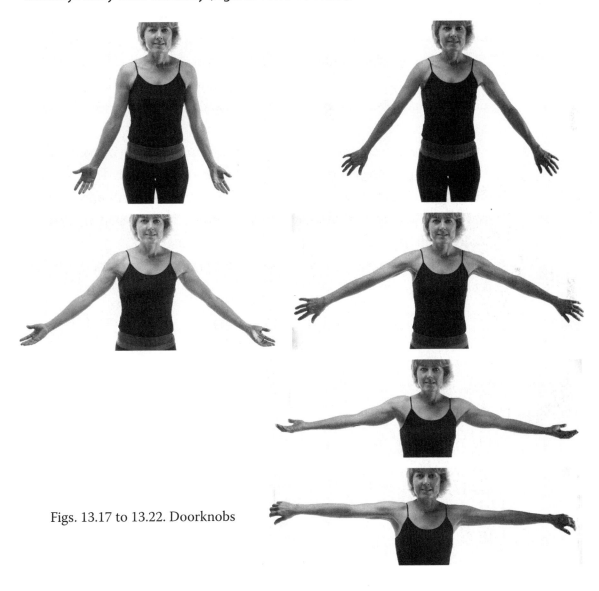

Figs. 13.17 to 13.22. Doorknobs

A CHAIR OR SHELVES FOR THE SHOULDER //

For this set of exercises, choose the back of a chair or shelves that are just below shoulder height. Take time to explore variations to see which direction helps most to release your tension patterns.

➤ Sitting on the chair, bend one elbow and rest it on the back of the chair or on a shelf. Let your body lean back into the elbow as you consciously relax all the muscles in your neck and at the top of your shoulder. It is important that you allow the chair or shelf to support you so you can sense all the tensions relaxing from your arm and shoulder area. Notice the sensation of slight compression toward your shoulder joint from your elbow lean (Figure 13.23).

Now, change your position on the chair or toward the shelf to bring that support, relaxation, and gentle compression toward your shoulder joint from different angles. Experiment to find the best angles for comfort (Figures 13.24 and 13.25).

Of course, a friend can also help by gently supporting your arm in the release position and giving compression from the elbow up toward the shoulder. I have occasionally even used the car headrest, armrest, and door for positional support and something to lean into for compression and release during traffic jams.

Remember that the key is to really relax the arm, neck, and shoulder as you lean.

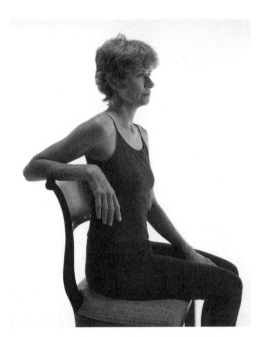

Fig. 13.23. Back to the "shelf"

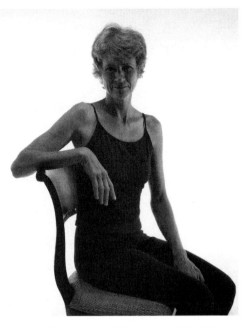

Fig. 13.24. Side to the "shelf"

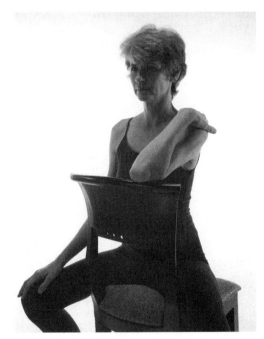

Fig. 13.25. Front to the "shelf"

Figs. 13.23 to 13.25. Positional variations for the shoulder "shelf" releases

※※※

Eight Shoulder Points with Specific Release Positions

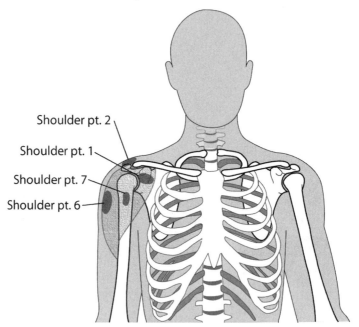

Fig. 13.26. Anterior shoulder points

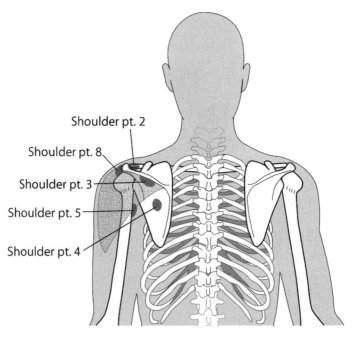

Fig. 13.27. Posterior shoulder points

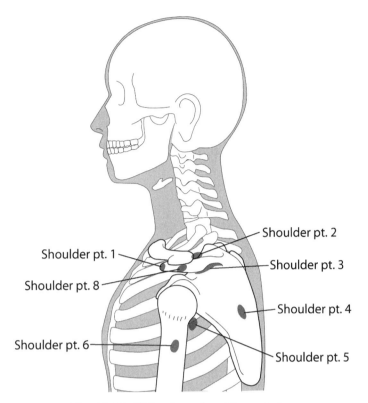

Fig. 13.28. Side view, shoulder points

The muscle groups comprising the shoulder allow the arm to move in several different directions. Because the shoulder area is complex, it releases more easily when you address one muscle group at a time. In Ortho-Bionomy there are eight specific shoulder positions that release eight specific indicator points. Tenderness at any one of these eight points indicates the corresponding position to use for release. Releasing these eight points with the matching position will release all the major muscle groups of the shoulder.

In these as in all the positional releases in this book it is important to remember to move slowly and fine-tune for just the right position. The tendency is to inadvertently skip over the release position in one's hurried efforts to deal with the pain. So go slowly, keeping your attention focused on your sensation, and feel for just the right position that brings relief from tension and pain. One of the ways to know if you are in the right position is to check the indicator point for tenderness. In the correct release position for your shoulder, the indicator point will not feel tender.

The position may be more effective if compression is applied from the elbow in toward the shoulder joint. So find a wall and lean into it.

Shoulder Point 1: Memory Point

Location

Although the shoulder blade (scapula) is in the back, it has a nose-like protrusion that extends forward to the front of the body just under the collarbone (clavicle) next to the top of your arm bone (humerus). This protrusion is called the coracoid process and is the location of the first shoulder indicator point (Figure 13.29). When there is tenderness or pain on or around this bone, use the following release position to relax the corresponding muscle group.

This point is also referred to as a "memory point" and can be rubbed for a few seconds during tests and examinations to help jog the memory. I once worked with a man in his nineties who had lived a very colorful life. During our sessions together he would tell some great stories, but usually somewhere in the story line he would forget what he was saying. One day as he lapsed into silence at a particularly interesting part, I reached over and rubbed his memory point (coracoid process) and he took right up where he had left off and finished his story. His wife's curiosity was immediately sparked. "How did you do that?" she asked. The memory point is one we can all use—it can also come in handy while studying for and taking a test!

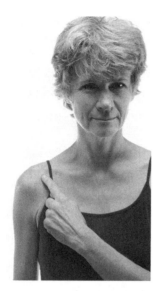

Fig. 13.29. Shoulder Point 1

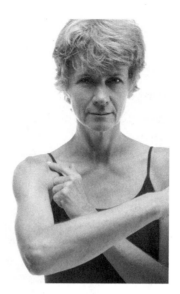

Fig. 13.30. Release position for Shoulder Point 1: The Cape

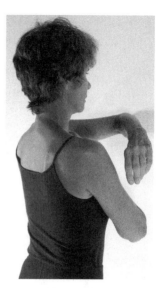

Fig. 13.31. Lean elbow into wall for compression from elbow into shoulder

RELEASE FOR SHOULDER POINT 1: THE CAPE //

➤ Standing, bend your elbow and bring your forearm up across your face into a comfortable position. My students often refer to this position as "The Cape" because the movement is one of drawing a cape around the front of your face (Figure 13.30).

If lying down in this position, get comfortable and allow your arm to relax and maintain this position for about two minutes. Sometimes applying a bit of compression from the elbow into the shoulder joint will release the tension more quickly. In this case, you may use your other arm to lightly push the elbow toward the shoulder.

If standing, swing the imaginary cape across your face, bringing your forearm up and across. Then lean your elbow into the wall, sensing the compression moving up from the elbow into the shoulder joint and slightly pushing the shoulder back (Figure 13.31).

Note any softening, pulsing, or reduced tenderness at the coracoid process.

※※※

Shoulder Point 2

Location

The indicator point for this position is in the narrow part of the sideways "V" (<) between the collarbone and the shoulder blade, on the top of the shoulder (Figure 13.32).

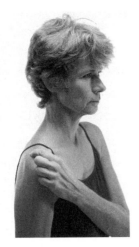

Fig. 13.32. Shoulder Point 2

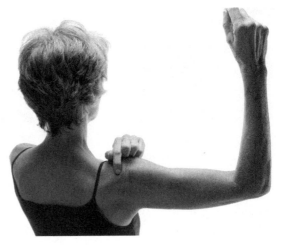

Fig. 13.33. Release position for Shoulder Point 2: arm at right angle

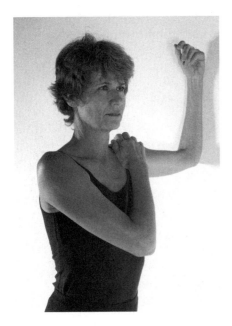

Fig. 13.34. Lean elbow into wall for compression into shoulder

RELEASE FOR SHOULDER POINT 2 ,,

➤ Standing with the wall to your side, raise your elbow out to shoulder height, making a right angle between your upper arm and your torso. Lean your elbow into the wall (Figures 13.33 to 13.34).

Sense the slight compression pushing gently from the elbow, through the upper arm into the shoulder joint. Remember to relax all the muscles at the shoulder and lower neck as you lean into the wall.

For maximum effectiveness, combine this with the 1st Rib Release.

%%%

Shoulder Point 3

Location

Shoulder Point 3 is actually a line of points located under the bony ridge that is the top edge of the scapula (Figure 13.35). If there is pain or tenderness under this ridge (spine of your scapula), use the following position to release.

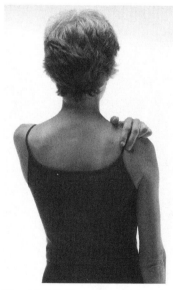

Fig. 13.35. Shoulder Point 3

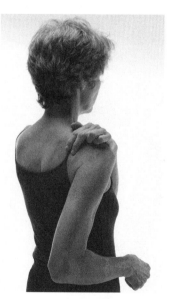

Fig. 13.36. Release position for Shoulder Point 3: Chicken Wing

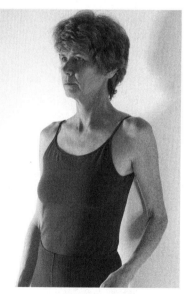

Fig. 13.37. Lean into wall for compression into shoulder

RELEASE FOR SHOULDER POINT 3: CHICKEN WING ⟫⟫⟫⟫⟫⟫⟫⟫⟫⟫⟫⟫⟫⟫⟫⟫⟫⟫⟫⟫⟫⟫

➤ Stand with your back to the wall, bend your elbow directly back (like a chicken wing), and lean your elbow into the wall. Keep your torso straight so the elbow lean creates a light compression from the elbow to the shoulder joint (Figures 13.36 to 13.37).

※※※

Shoulder Point 4

Location

The indicator for Shoulder Point 4 is located in the middle of the scapula. You can find the midpoint of someone else's scapula by placing your thumb and forefinger under the lower "V" of the shoulder bone. The indicator point will be midway between your thumb and forefinger. You can reach back under or over your own arm and check the point in the middle of the scapula (Figures 13.38 to 13.40).

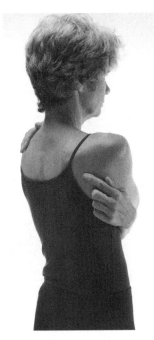

Fig. 13.38. Shoulder Point 4

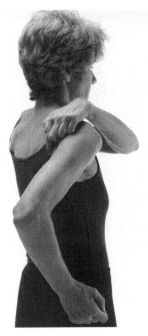

Fig. 13.39. Release position for Shoulder Point 4: Turkey Wing

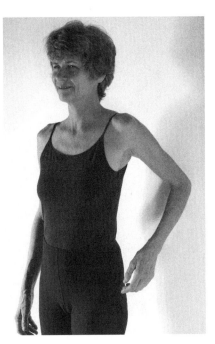

Fig. 13.40. Lean into wall for compression toward shoulder

RELEASE FOR SHOULDER POINT 4: TURKEY WING ,,,

➤ Standing with your back to the wall, bend your elbow back and slightly to the side. Note that in this position your elbow is slightly to the side rather than straight back as above—we call this position the Turkey Wing to differentiate it from the Chicken Wing position that releases Shoulder Point 3. Lean your elbow into the wall. Stabilize the torso so the elbow lean creates compression back toward the shoulder joint (Figures 13.39 and 13.40).

‰‰‰

Shoulder Point 5

Location

Shoulder Point 5 is another short series of points found on the back of the arm or the torso on either side of the armpit crease. Any tender point along either side of the upside-down "V" made by the arm and torso at the back of the armpit is an indicator to use the following release position (Figure 13.40).

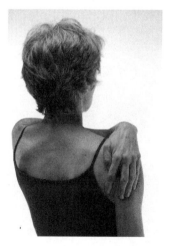

Fig. 13.41. Shoulder Point 5

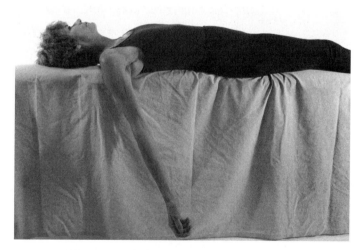

Fig. 13.42. Release position
for Shoulder Point 5: Arm Drop

RELEASE FOR SHOULDER POINT 5: ARM DROP ,,,

➤ Lie on your back on a bed or couch near the edge, and drop your arm down toward the floor. Rotate your arm so the palm faces the ceiling. If this position is comfortable and doesn't create any strain in your shoulder, allow your arm to hang there for a minute or so and completely relax (Figure 13.42).

If it feels more comfortable, place a chair with a pillow on it to support the arm as it hangs in the release position.

Slowly and gently return your arm to your side.

%%%

Shoulder Point 6

Location

Shoulder Point 6 is located on the side of your arm in the muscle group about where a very short sleeve would fall. It is in the center of the belly of the deltoid muscle (Figure 13.43). This point corresponds to pain when the elbow lifts up and out from the body at a right angle. *Often in shoulder injuries, this is the last point to clear and the last movement to give up its pain—so be patient and continue with this release over time.*

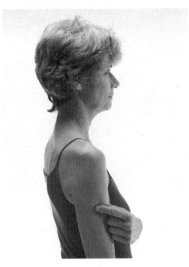

Fig. 13.43. Shoulder Point 6

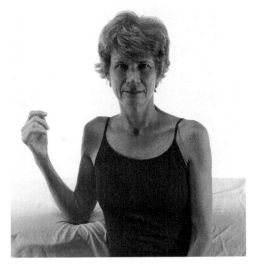

Fig. 13.44. Release position for Shoulder Point 6. Lean into elbow for compression into shoulder.

RELEASE FOR SHOULDER POINT 6 ,,

➤ Sitting with your arm next to a table, bend your elbow and rest it on the table with your palm facing forward and up. Be sure to keep your body close to the elbow. Lean into the elbow for compression toward your shoulder joint (Figure 13.44).

If you place your finger very lightly on the indicator point, you may feel a subtle pulsing or softening under your fingertip.

※※※

Shoulder Point 7

Location

Shoulder Point 7 is another short series of points located on the front of the upper arm, on the humerus itself, next to the armpit crease (Figure 13.45).

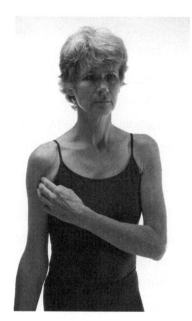
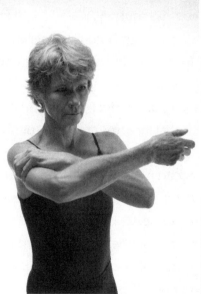
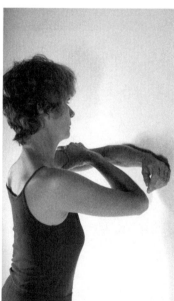

Fig. 13.45. Shoulder Point 7

Fig. 13.46. Release position for Shoulder Point 7

Fig. 13.47. Lean into wall for compression toward shoulder

RELEASE FOR SHOULDER POINT 7 ,,,

➤ Stand facing a wall. Place the thumb of the opposite hand gently on the indicator point, and grasp the tender affected upper arm in your hand. Roll the skin and muscle of the upper arm in toward the armpit.

Still holding the flesh rolled, bend the elbow of your affected arm and raise it into a comfortable position across your face. Then turn that hand toward your face (Figure 13.46).

Maintain this position as you lean the elbow of the affected arm into the wall, creating compression from the elbow toward the shoulder joint (Figure 13.47).

ISOTONIC RELEASE FOR SHOULDER POINT 7:
HITCHHIKING OUT OF THE CAPE ,,

Movement against resistance, an isotonic exercise, balances muscle tone and often relieves pain quickly; it works well for this point. See Chapter 1 for general information about isotonic exercises.

My twenty-four-year-old daughter had been complaining of a sore arm and asked for a session. After we released all the arm and shoulder points, she still was feeling discomfort. I showed her this isotonic exercise to tone, strengthen, and rebalance the muscles throughout her range of motion. Doing this exercise finally released her pain. Repeating this exercise frequently helps to reeducate and strengthen more effective and functional muscle use.

➤ The set up for this isotonic is the same as the position of release: Place the thumb of the opposite hand on the indicator point, grasp the top of the sore upper arm, and roll the muscle toward the armpit. Bend the elbow and bring it to a comfortable position across your face, turning the palm of your hand toward your face (Figure 13.48).

Initiate a "hitchhiking" movement from the thumb of your affected arm to bring the hand across the front like a windshield wiper while your other hand holding the rolled upper arm maintains a slight resistance to the movement (Figure 13.49).

Allow the upper arm to gradually and smoothly roll through the resistance of your grasp (Figures 13.50 and 13.51).

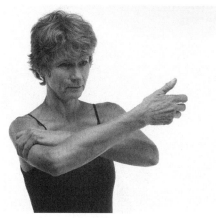

Fig. 13.48. Rotate upper arm toward point and bring hand in front of face

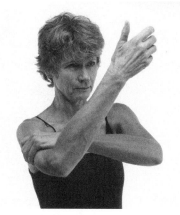

Fig. 13.49. Begin to move arm against resistance of grasp

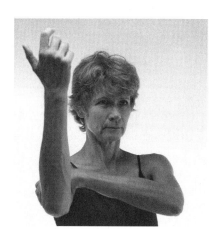

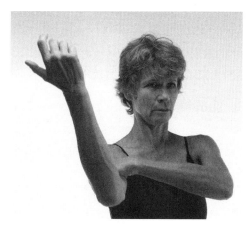

Figs. 13.50 and 13.51. Thumb leads arm across face against resistance of upper arm grasp

Figs. 13.48 to 13.51. Isotonic Release for Shoulder Point 7: Hitchhiking Out of the Cape

※※※

Shoulder Point 8

Location

The indicator point for this position is located on the outside edge of the shoulder joint, at the outside notch where the clavicle and scapula meet (Figure 13.52).

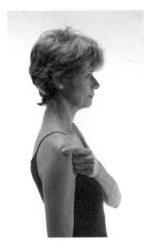

Fig. 13.52. Shoulder Point 8

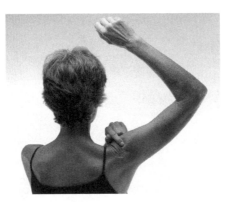

Fig. 13.53. Release position for Shoulder Point 8

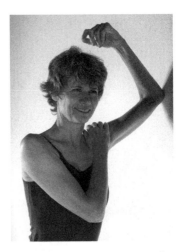

Fig. 13.54. Lean into wall for compression into shoulder

RELEASE FOR SHOULDER POINT 8 ,,

➤ Standing with your affected side next to the wall, bend your elbow and raise your arm sideways above shoulder height. Lean your elbow into the wall, applying compression back toward the shoulder joint (Figure 13.53 and 13.54).

※※※

Isometrics to Release Shoulders

In an attempt to avoid pain, the body often limits movement by constricting and contracting surrounding muscles. Then fear of pain reinforces the holding. While immobilization may solve the pain problem in the moment, it can set up compensatory tension and holding patterns that limit movement and optimal function.

We use isometric movement in Ortho-Bionomy Self-Care to prompt the nervous system to reestablish normal movement and function. An isometric against resistance educates and empowers us to move through restrictive patterning.

These next exercises are beneficial for interrupting holding patterns that block relaxed and naturally integrated functional movement in the shoulders. They can be very effective for frozen shoulder.

When using isometric or isotonic exercises, always start by finding the most comfortable position. From this position, you'll initiate movement against the resistance—in this case, a wall—to interrupt the tension pattern. Working with the shoulder, you'll initiate the movement from the lower arm and elbow, not from the torso.

At the end of each isometric exercise it is important to follow through with the movement you were attempting, so the muscle senses a completion of the movement.

BACK TO THE WALL, ELBOW AT SIDE

You may do this exercise with both elbows at the same time to awaken the body's memory of upright posture. This can be an especially effective technique for the elderly.

➤ Stand with your back to the wall, elbow bent at your side and your hand extending forward.

Slightly push your elbow straight back into the wall for ten seconds while you visualize the elbow moving through the wall (Figure 13.55).

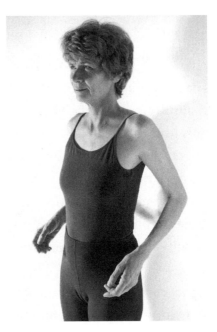

Fig. 13.55. Push against wall

Release the resistance as you step away from the wall and allow the elbow to continue to follow through the attempted movement. This relaxed follow-through completes the movement you were attempting in the isometric (Figure 13.56).

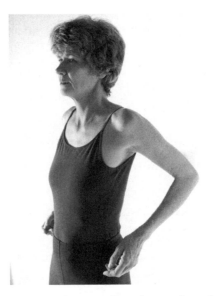

Fig. 13.56. Step away from wall and complete the movement

SIDE TO THE WALL, ELBOW AT SIDE,,,

➤ Stand with the wall to your side, your elbow bent at your side and your hand extending forward.

Push your lower arm and elbow into the wall for ten seconds and then release (Figure 13.57).

Step away from the wall and allow the elbow to rise sideways and up to complete the movement you were attempting to make (Figure 13.58).

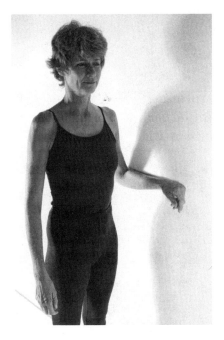

Fig. 13.57. Push lower arm into wall

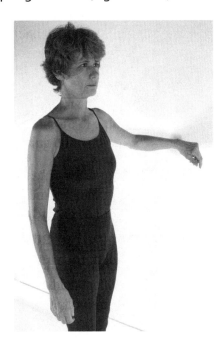

Fig. 13.58. Step away from wall and complete the movement

SIDE TO THE WALL, ELBOW IN FRONT AT SHOULDER HEIGHT ⁄⁄⁄⁄⁄⁄⁄⁄⁄⁄⁄⁄⁄⁄⁄⁄⁄⁄

➤ Stand next to the wall with your elbow at shoulder level and forearm across the front of your body.

Push your elbow and back of upper arm against the wall for ten seconds while imagining that the arm is moving effortlessly through the wall (Figure 13.59).

After ten seconds, step away from the wall and allow the elbow and arm to swing back in the direction it had been attempting to move and then forward again (Figure 13.60).

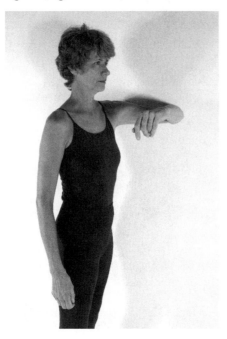

Fig. 13.59. Push upper arm into wall

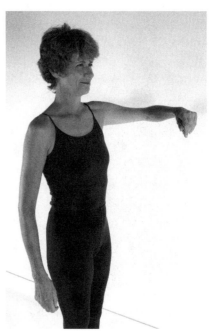

Fig. 13.60. Step away from wall and swing elbow back and forth

FACING THE WALL, ELBOW AT WAIST ,,,

➤ Face the wall, bend your elbow, and rest your forearm in front of your body at waist level, palm down.

Push the back of your forearm into the wall, imagining an arc that your arm would make away from your torso and up toward your face (Figure 13.61).

Push for ten seconds and then release. Move away from the wall and complete the arc movement you were visualizing (Figure 13.62).

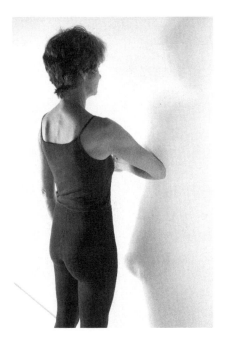

Fig. 13.61. Push lower arm into wall

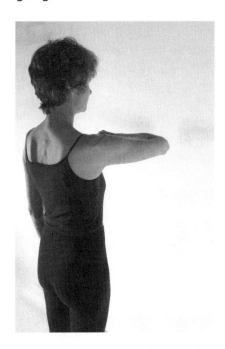

Fig. 13.62. Step away from wall and complete the movement

CHAPTER 14

Arms, Elbows, Wrists, and Hands

Arms and hands enable physical expression, allowing us to reach out for what we want, pull it in for a closer look, or push it away if disagreeable. They can spring to action to protect and defend or just as easily embrace a friend. We use them to communicate when we wave and gesture or use very specific hand and finger movements to "speak" with the deaf. Through our sense of touch we discover and soothe, measure and describe, and, if blind, read and orient.

The shoulders, arms, elbows, wrists, and hands working together provide a wide range of mobility and flexibility. Large encompassing movements as well as fine motor skills are coordinated by the interaction of muscles and nerves. Sensory (feeling) and motor (movement) nerves carry impulses back and forth from the spinal cord to the many muscle groups, allowing us to accomplish an incredible variety of tasks. We can type with speed and accuracy, as well as coordinate the movements of a golf swing with grace and precision. We can accurately throw a ball or thread a needle.

The functioning of one neighborhood can affect the functionality of another—tension in the shoulder and neck muscles can create pain in the hand or elbow. Recognizing the interrelationships among the spine, shoulders, arms, elbows, wrists, and hands helps us to become more aware of the importance of addressing all the neighborhoods. We thereby deal more effectively with tension, pain, and discomfort.

Anatomy of the Brachial Plexus

A network of nerves, the brachial (arm) plexus, originates between the last four vertebrae in the neck, crosses over the front of the shoulder and under the collarbone, then branches out and extends to various muscles throughout the arm and hand (Figure 14.1).

Anywhere along its path, tensions can impinge effective functioning, leading to impaired movement or any number of sensations, such as dull aches in the arm or tingling in the fingers. Interweaving through several neighborhoods, this network of nerves demonstrates the interconnectedness of the neck, shoulder, ribs, arm, wrist, and hand. This is why we work with all the adjacent areas, so the neighbors maintain flexible and functional relationships with one another. The 1st Rib Release (Chapter 12) is a great place to begin since it is at a key intersection of the neck, shoulder, and ribs.

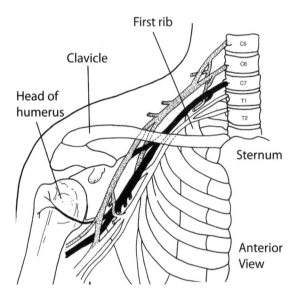

Fig. 14.1. Brachial plexus. Courtesy of *Illustrated Essentials of Musculoskeletal Anatomy,* 4th Edition, by Sieg and Adams (Gainesville, FL: Megabooks, Inc., 1992), www.muscleanatomybook.com.

Release Positions for the Arms

Tenderness at either of these anterior (front) or posterior (back) indicator points can signify poor circulation throughout shoulder, arm, and hand.

Include both of these releases any time you have discomfort in the arm. Work with one point at a time, gently positioning around it for comfort.

Often symptoms of pain in the arm, hand, and shoulder occur during menopause, suggesting an endocrine correlation. Remember to use the releases for the rotated hips and pelvis in Chapter 3 when there is an endocrine imbalance. Also see Chapter 20 for more release positions for nerve pain in the arm.

RELEASE POSITION FOR FRONT ARM INDICATOR POINTS: CROSS PULL ,,,,,,,,

Indicator points for tenderness or poor circulation of the arm are located on the outside (lateral) edge of the upper chest, just below where the arm attaches to the torso. This means they are found at the pectoralis minor muscle attachments on the 3rd, 4th, and 5th ribs (Figures 14.2 and 14.3).

➤ Gently grasp above the elbow on the affected side and slowly pull your affected arm across your body, making a cave around the points to ease the tenderness. Release the pull and maintain relaxation in the positioned crossed arm; recheck the point for release (Figure 14.4). Hold the position for ten to twenty seconds.

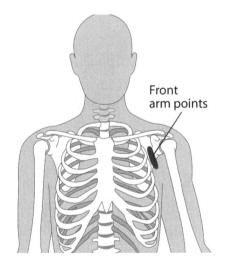

Fig. 14.2. Front arm points

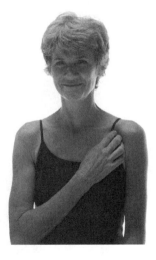

Fig. 14.3. Finding front arm points

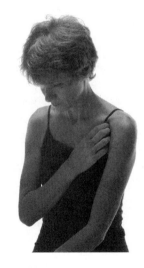

Fig. 14.4. Crossed arm release

RELEASE POSITION FOR POSTERIOR ARM POINTS: "UNCLE" OR "I GIVE UP"

Posterior (back) points for arm pain are located along the upper, inner (medial) edge of the scapula at the level of the 1st, 2nd, and 3rd ribs (Figures 14.5 and 14.6).

➤ Bring the affected arm behind your back and bend the affected elbow. Bring your other hand behind your back to lightly grasp the wrist of the affected arm and gently pull the elbow across your body toward the unaffected side. No need to "cry uncle," but it can prove beneficial to think about surrendering and releasing the front of the shoulder joint. Hold this position for ten to thirty seconds (Figure 14.7).

Keep in mind:

For hard-to-release arm pain, you may need to use the release positions for the neck, upper back, and 1st rib, as well as those for the shoulder, arm, elbow, and wrist.

Tension and pain in the upper arm is generally relieved with the shoulder release positions and exercises, especially the Shoulder Point 6 release and the Hitchhiking isotonic of Shoulder Point 7. Arm releases are also included in Chapter 20.

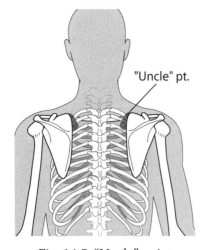

Fig. 14.5. "Uncle" point

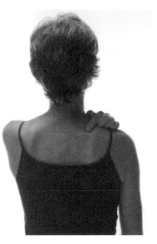

Fig. 14.6. Find the "Uncle" point

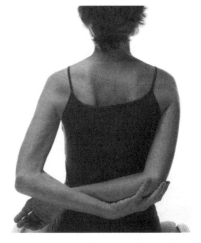

Fig. 14.7. Release position for scapula

※※※

Elbow

Because it is the joint "in the middle"—between the wrist and the shoulder—the elbow experiences particular types of stresses. Just as the knee modulates movement from the ankle and hip, the elbow is the mediator between tensions in the shoulder and the wrist. Remember its neighbors when working with the elbow: begin with releasing the shoulder and wrist, and then do the releases for the elbow. This is especially important for "tennis elbow."

Isotonic movements with the elbow release can also be key to effectively rebalancing muscle tone in the lower arm and reducing elbow discomfort and pain.

Anatomy

The elbow is a hinge joint, formed by the connection of the bone of the upper arm (humerus) to the bones of the lower arm (the radius and the ulna). The radius is the bone on the thumb side of the arm; the ulna is on the little-finger side. A strong ligament at the elbow joint wraps around the head of the radius. This ligament and the inter-osseous membrane between the two forearm bones support rotational movement, allowing the radius to roll over the top of the ulna to turn the palm up (Figure 14.8).

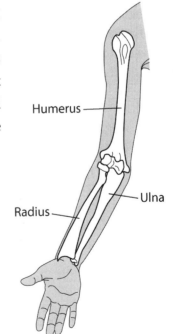

Humerus

Ulna

Radius

Fig. 14.8. Anatomy of the elbow

Positional Releases and Isometric Exercises for the Elbow

FLEXION AND EXTENSION RELEASE ,,,

This exercise could also be called "Start Where You Are and Compress." I was once called to the hospital bedside of a friend who had been in a car accident. She was in what is called a waking coma, sitting up with eyes open but not seemingly present. Her limbs were tightly contracted so I took her hand in mine and began adding compression from her hand toward her wrist. The nurse came in to take her blood pressure and began to struggle with the intense muscle contractures as she attempted to straighten the elbow. I suggested to the nurse that instead of fighting the contracture, she could compress down the line of the bone from the wrist toward the elbow joint. She tried it and my friend's elbow immediately extended. As the nurse looked at me with surprise, I assured her that she could use this with anyone with tight muscle contractions. It is always good to remember the simple principles of this work when faced with muscular tension.

➤ First, see if the elbow bends (flexes) and straightens (extends) easily and completely.

If there is resistance to bending or straightening, start with the elbow in a position where you feel comfortable.

Rest your bent elbow in the comfortable position on a table. Hold on to the wrist with your other hand and gently press the forearm down toward the elbow to create compression for ten to thirty seconds (Figure 14.9).

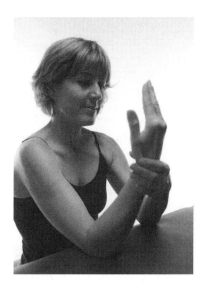

Fig. 14.9. Add compression from wrist toward elbow

⁂

Isometrics to Increase Range of Motion

An isometric will encourage further range of motion. You may repeat these isometric exercises every couple of hours throughout the day to gently remind the body of its capacity for increased movement.

Remember that the body may only accept a small amount of change at a time. Don't work hard or aim for big change; you will get better results by working slowly and consistently, allowing the body to integrate in its own time. Sometimes it may seem as if we are only dropping pebbles, but at some point the body can spontaneously organize those pebbles into a path.

ISOMETRIC TO INCREASE FLEXION (BENDING)⸝⸝⸝⸝⸝⸝⸝⸝⸝⸝⸝⸝⸝⸝⸝⸝⸝⸝⸝⸝⸝⸝⸝⸝⸝⸝⸝⸝⸝⸝⸝⸝⸝⸝⸝⸝⸝⸝

➤ Once again, with your elbow resting on the table, bend the elbow only as far as it moves easily and comfortably. With your other hand, apply gentle resistance to the inside of the wrist while you attempt to bend your elbow more. The resisting hand prevents movement but does not overwhelm the attempted movement. A small amount of resistance that just meets the amount of attempted movement is most useful.

Be sure to visualize your arm moving in the direction of the attempted movement.

Hold the gentle resistance for only ten seconds and then release and follow through. Check to see if the elbow has a greater capacity for flexion by slowly and passively moving the arm through flexion and extension with your other hand. Notice if the range of motion has increased (Figures 14.10 and 14.11).

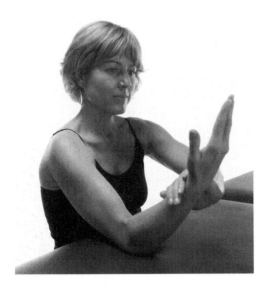

Fig. 14.10. Apply resistance while attempting to bend the elbow more

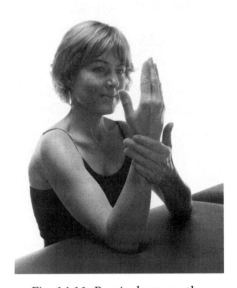

Fig. 14.11. Passively move the arm to complete the attempted movement

ISOMETRIC TO INCREASE EXTENSION (STRAIGHTENING)˒˒˒˒˒˒˒˒˒˒˒˒˒˒˒˒˒˒˒˒˒˒˒˒˒˒˒˒

➤ If the elbow resists complete extension, bend to the position of comfort and rest your elbow on the table. With your other hand, apply gentle resistance to the back of the wrist as you attempt to straighten the arm. The resisting hand prevents movement but does not overwhelm the attempted movement. A small amount of resistance that just meets the amount of attempted movement is most useful (Figure 14.12).

Remember to visualize yourself completing the movement you are attempting.

Hold the gentle resistance for only ten seconds and then release and follow through. Check to see if the elbow has a greater capacity for extension (Figure 14.13).

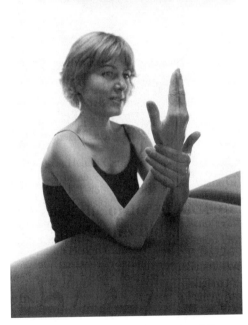

Fig. 14.12. Apply resistance while attempting to straighten arm

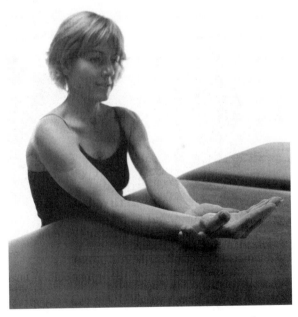

Fig. 14.13. Passively move arm to complete attempted movement

※※※

Tender Elbow Points

You may find that there are sore or tender points located around the heads of the bones of the elbow. Check for tenderness on both sides of the arm just above the elbow and below the elbow at the heads of the humerus, the radius, and the ulna (Figures 14.14 to 14.16).

You can also check for tenderness or tension in the muscle and tissue between the bones.

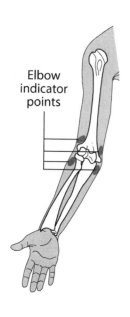

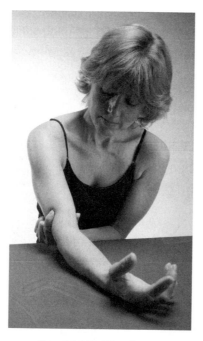

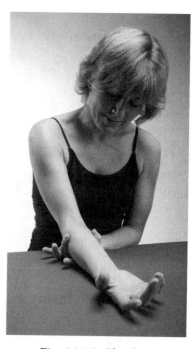

Fig. 14.14. Elbow points

Fig. 14.15. Check for tenderness above elbow joint

Fig. 14.16. Check for tenderness below elbow joint

RELEASING TENDER ELBOW POINTS

Focus on one tender spot at a time.

➤ Bend the elbow, resting it on a table so your hand is in the air. With your other hand rotate the forearm in one direction and check the tender point, and then rotate the forearm in the other direction and compare tenderness now.

Rotate the forearm whichever way reduces the tenderness of the point, and compress the forearm toward the elbow joint. Hold the position and compression for ten to thirty seconds (Figures 14.17 to 14.19).

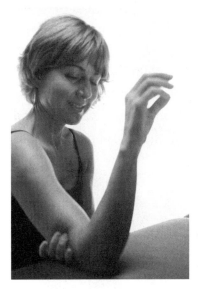
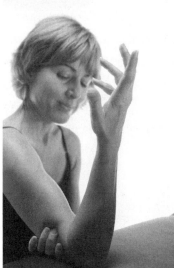
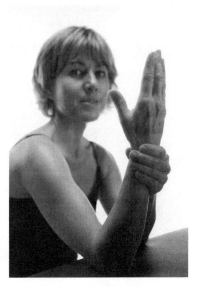

Fig. 14.17. Rotate wrist and then check point for tenderness

Fig. 14.18. Rotate wrist in opposite direction and recheck point

Fig. 14.19. Rotate wrist toward direction of less tenderness and compress from wrist toward elbow

ISOMETRIC AND ISOTONIC EXERCISES
TO RELEASE TENDER INDICATOR POINTS

Often it is more effective to use an isometric or isotonic exercise to address a painful elbow and to release tension between the bones of the lower arm. An isotonic is especially useful when the tension and tenderness are caused by unbalanced muscle tone.

➤ As in the above positioning, rotate the forearm to the position that reduces the tenderness at the point (Figure 14.20). Grasp the wrist or forearm with your other hand and provide gentle resistance while attempting to rotate out of the position (Figure 14.21).

If you choose to do an isometric, apply just enough resistance to meet the effort of the rotating arm so the arm does not rotate at all. If you choose to try an isotonic, apply just enough resistance to allow the arm to slowly rotate within your grasp. An isometric (no rotation allowed) usually increases ease and range of motion; the isotonic (allowing movement) helps to release tension and tone the muscles of the forearm. Be sensitive to the amount of pressure of the resistance. Don't overpower the effort. You want the muscles to work but not to strain.

After holding resistance for seven to ten seconds, allow the rotation efforts to follow through and complete the movement (Figures 14.22 and 14.23).

Experiment with all three types of release—compression, isometric, and isotonic—to see which gives the greatest release at the tender point.

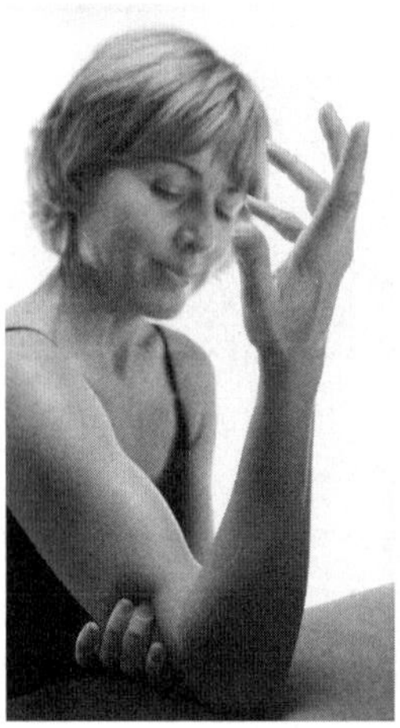

Fig. 14.20. Rotate wrist and then check point for tenderness

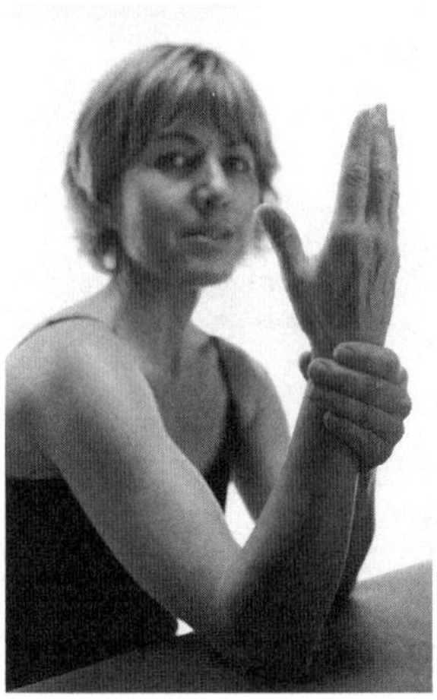

Fig. 14.21. Apply resistance to allow slight slow rotation of wrist

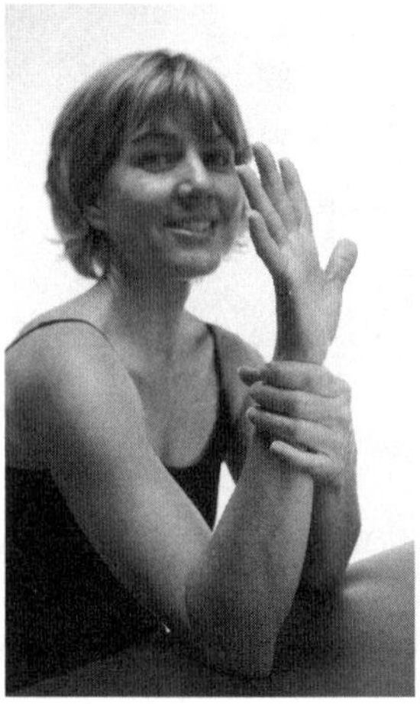

Fig. 14.22. Complete attempted movement

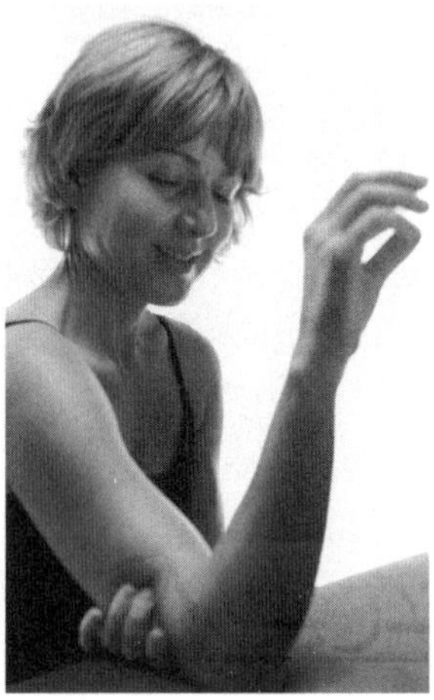

Fig. 14.23. Recheck point

Wrists and Hands: Anatomy

The wrist joint consists of the two bones of the forearm (the radius at the thumb side and the ulna at the little-finger side) meeting with the first of two rows of the eight small metacarpal bones of the hand. The wrist allows for flexion and extension (bye-bye wave), abduction and adduction (lateral movements toward the thumb and toward the little finger, like a flat-handed wave), and circular rotations of the wrist and hand (Figure 14.24).

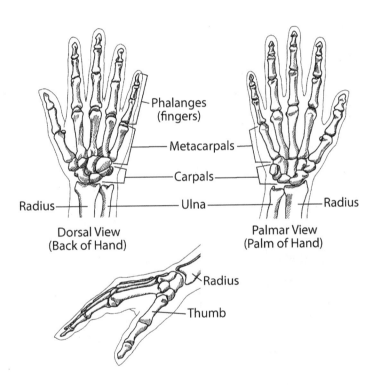

Fig. 14.24. Anatomy of the wrist and hand

Release Positions for the Wrist

The wrists and fingers can get sprained or strained from injury or overuse, or they might be tight and sore from arthritis. The positional release techniques offered below can reduce inflammation, pain, and tenderness in these areas.

All of the following release positions call for compression back toward the wrist from the hand. Remember to do the assessments, positioning, and compression slowly and gently.

FLEXION/EXTENSION

➤ Bend your wrist into flexion, curling the palm toward the wrist. Then move the wrist back into extension, moving the back of the hand toward the forearm. Feel which position is more comfortable. With your other hand, take the hand into the position of most comfort and gently compress from the hand in toward the wrist. Hold for ten seconds (Figures 14.25 to 14.27).

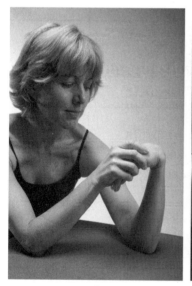
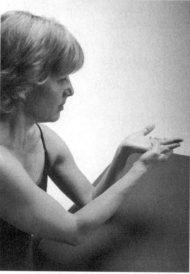
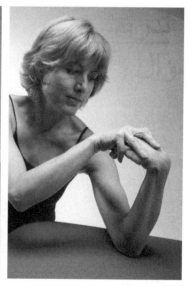

Fig. 14.25. Wrist flexion

Fig. 14.26. Wrist extension

Fig. 14.27. Compress in preferred position toward wrist

LATER AL BENDING///

➤ Laterally bend the wrist, bringing the thumb and wrist closer together, and then bend the wrist in the opposite direction, taking the little finger toward the wrist (like an old-fashioned clock's pendulum). Again note which position is more comfortable. With your other hand, take the hand into the position of most comfort and gently compress from the hand toward the wrist (Figures 14.28 and 14.29). Hold for ten seconds.

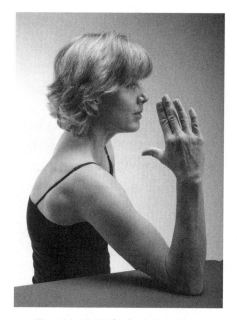

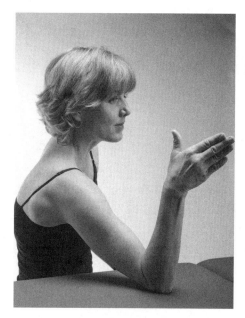

Fig. 14.28. Side-bend wrist to thumb side

Fig. 14.29. Side-bend wrist toward the little finger

WRITE WRIST ROTATION //

➤ Rest your elbow on a table in front of you. Rotate your wrist, first with the palm toward the face and then with the palm away from the face, noting the direction that feels most comfortable. Rotate again to the most comfortable position, then gently grasp the hand and compress from the hand in toward the wrist (Figures 14.30 to 14.32). Hold for ten seconds.

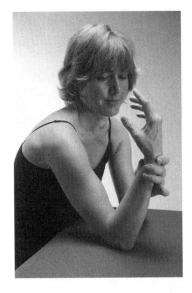

Fig. 14.30. Rotate palm toward face

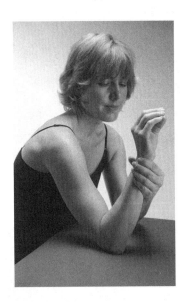

Fig. 14.31. Rotate palm away from face

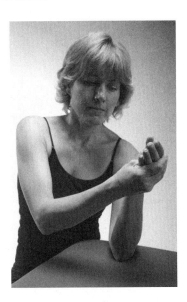

Fig. 14.32. Compress in preferred position toward wrist

WRIST CIRCLES //

➤ Slowly rotate the wrist in a circle, feeling for places of tension, pain, or discomfort, or a glitch or resistance in the movement (Figures 14.33 to 14.39).

Then move the wrist to a position directly across from the glitch, discomfort, or resistance. You may also move the wrist to a position in the rotation just before the tension.

With your other hand, gently compress the hand toward the wrist (Figure 14.40). Hold the compression for ten seconds.

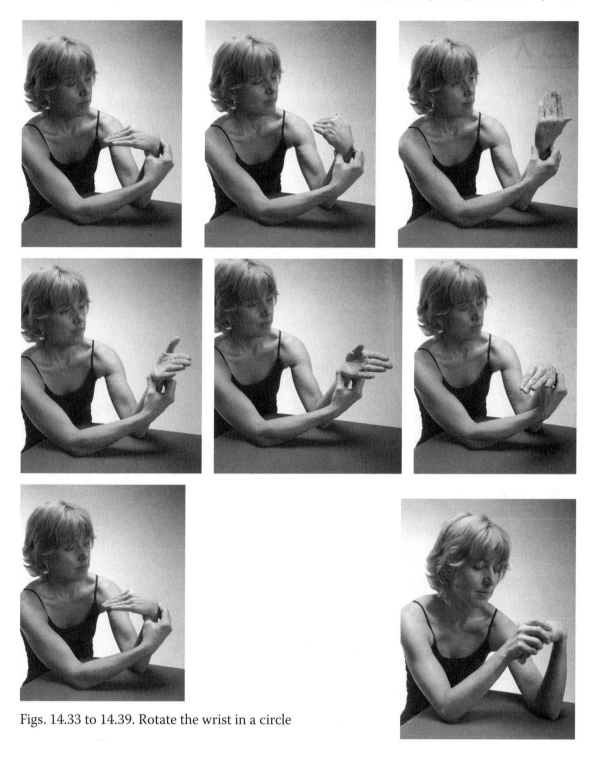

Figs. 14.33 to 14.39. Rotate the wrist in a circle

Fig. 14.40. Compress toward wrist just before the "glitch"

BRACELET POINTS ,,,

➤ Press gently around the wrist, including the heads of the carpal bones, feeling for tender points or tension. When you find a tender place, gently curl the hand around the tender point in such a way as to reduce the pain. This curl may include a slight rotation of the hand to get to just the right angle for you. Add gentle compression from the hand toward the wrist, for ten seconds, then release back to a neutral position (Figures 14.41 to 14.43).

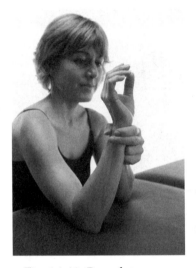

Fig. 14.41. Bracelet points

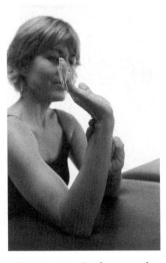

Fig. 14.42. Curl around tender point

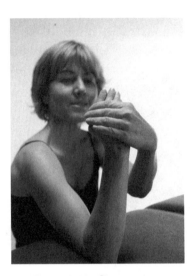

Fig. 14.43. Compress toward wrist

⁒⁒⁒

Hand

The hand is designed to be dexterous and skillful, strong and sensitive, with the capacity for grasping, gripping, and pushing as well as very fine-tuned motor movement.

I have spent full one-hour sessions on just the fingers and hands of violinists and other musicians. One woman who plays violin has begun to get arthritis in her hands. These gentle rotations and compressions into each joint of each finger have helped to release her pain and stiffness and increased her ability to maintain flexibility and dexterity.

The hand consists of the eight small carpal bones, five long bones called metacarpals that connect the carpal bones to the fingers, and the fourteen phalanges or individual bones of the fingers and thumb (Figure 14.44).

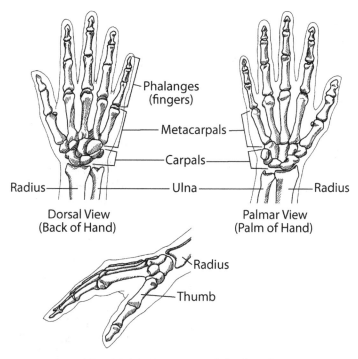

Fig. 14.44. Anatomy of the hand

Releases for the Hand and Fingers

Tension or torque can occur at each of the many joints of the hand; you can release each of the joints by positioning for greatest comfort and adding compression.

Take time to fully explore and determine the positional relationship between the two bones that are uncomfortable. This exploration allows you to sense the direction of the holding and to compress into the area in a way that slightly shortens the tight muscles and takes the internal tension off the area. This might involve squeezing two of the long bones of the hand closer together or compressing from a finger back through the knuckle toward the hand. Be willing to experiment for the position that shortens tense muscles and brings relief.

Hold the compression into the area for ten to thirty seconds and then release, slowly and gently pulling out and away from the direction of compression and stretching the hand and fingers.

CHECK THE HAND FOR FLEXIBILITY AND TENDER POINTS ,,,,,,,,,,,,,,,,,,,,,,,,,,,,,,

➤ Hold one hand in the other and, with the pad of your thumb, gently palpate and massage the palm of the held hand (Figures 14.45 and 14.47). What do you sense? Can you feel movement between the bones? Are there any tight spaces or places of tension between the bones? Does the hand flex (curl) and have springiness? Do you notice any tender points?

If you find a tender point, curl the hand around the tender point and gently squeeze the palm of the hand, bringing the thumb in toward the little finger (Figure 14.46). Hold the squeeze for ten to thirty seconds and then release. Palpate again and see if you sense any difference. You may need to try different angles of compression (Figure 14.48).

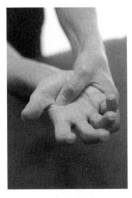
Fig. 14.45. Explore for tender points

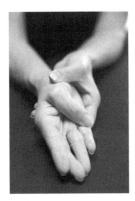
Fig. 14.46. Squeeze palm

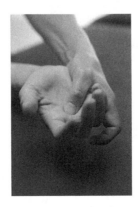
Fig. 14.47. Check for tender points

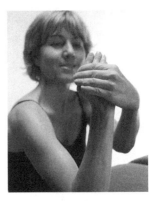
Fig. 14.48. Curl around tender point and compress

CHECKING AND INCREASING THE RANGE
OF MOTION IN THE FINGERS

➤ Check the ability of the fingers to extend (straighten) and flex (curl) toward the palm.

You may address all the fingers as a whole or one finger at a time. To address tightness or pain in a finger joint, simply bend the finger just as much as is comfortable and then gently compress from the end of the finger back toward the joint (Figure 14.49). If the finger joint feels better with a bit of rotation, then add a little rotation to the flexion before adding the compression (Figure 14.50). Hold the compression for ten to twenty seconds and then release by moving the finger around to explore greater range of motion.

If all the fingers prefer to flex, flex them all a bit more; with your other hand squeeze and compress them in the flexed position toward the hand, hold for ten to twenty seconds, and release (Figure 14.51). Then check to see if there is more extension available by moving the fingers passively to determine if the range of movement has increased.

For Dupuytren's contractures, in which the fingers are flexed and the palm of the hand is contracted and ridged, use the Release for Parker's Reflex in Chapter 20.

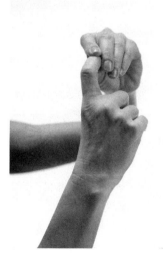

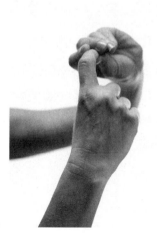

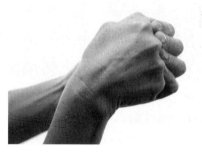

Fig. 14.51. Squeeze flexed fingers

Fig. 14.49. Compress into flexed finger joint

Fig. 14.50. Twist and compress toward joint

If your finger(s) seem stuck in flexion (curled), you can encourage extension using an isometric. Hold the finger in its most comfortable flexed position while you try to extend (straighten) it against your gentle resistance. Attempt to extend against the resistance for seven to ten seconds and release. After the isometric, follow through on the attempted movement by gently pulling the finger out (Figures 14.52 and 14.53).

Remember, when giving resistance, you don't want to overpower the joint; just give enough resistance for the finger to have something to push against.

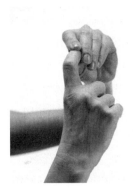

Fig. 14.52. Attempt to straighten finger against gentle resistance

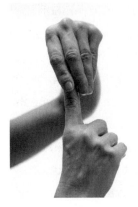

Fig. 14.53. Gently pull finger after isometric

RELEASING THE FINGERS

➤ If a finger or thumb does not flex (bend) comfortably, compress the phalange (finger bone) toward its nearest flexed joint. If the finger has a rotation preference, add that twist to the compression (Figure 14.54). Sometimes the bone on one side of the joint will want to rotate one direction while the bone on the other side will twist more easily to the opposite direction. Be sure to check the rotation preference of each joint. The more specifically you can match the preferences and angle of holding, the more successful you will be at releasing the tiny holding patterns around the joints.

If the finger flexes a little but will not curl into the palm, flex to where it is comfortable, then add compression into the nearest joint (Figure 14.55).

Repeat on each joint of the finger. After compression, encourage greater flexion by gently moving the finger toward the palm and then away.

You may also try an isometric. Hold the finger in its extended (straight) position and attempt to flex but don't allow any movement for seven to ten seconds, using your other hand to resist. After releasing the resistance, follow through the attempted movement by passively moving the finger to encourage better flexion (Figures 14.56 and 14.57). Remember to visualize the finger flexing as you are attempting the movement.

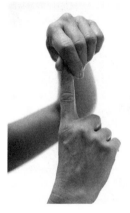

Fig. 14.54. Rotate and compress into the joints of a non-bending finger

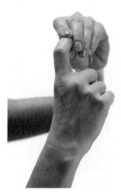

Fig. 14.55. Rotate and compress toward slightly flexed joint

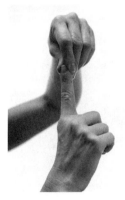

Fig. 14.56. Attempt to bend finger against slight resistance

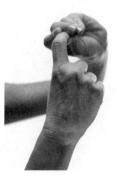

Fig. 14.57. After isometric gently encourage finger to bend

ROTATING THE FINGERS AND THUMBS

➤ Release individual fingers and joints by rotating or twisting each bone to where it feels most comfortable and then compressing the bone back toward the nearest joint (Figures 14.58 and 14.59). Sometimes the bone on one end of the joint will want to rotate one way, and the next bone will feel more comfortable twisting in the opposite direction. Simply address each joint individually by rotating in the preferred directions and compress toward the joint. Hold the compressions for ten to thirty seconds and release (Figures 14.60 to 14.62).

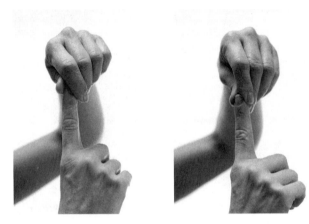

Figs. 14.58 and 14.59. Rotate and compress toward preference

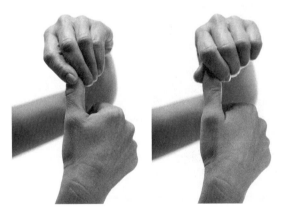

Figs. 14.60 and 14.61. Rotate the thumb

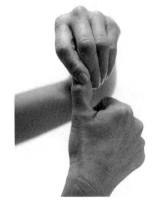

Fig. 14.62. Rotate to preference and compress toward slightly flexed joint

RELEASE FOR THE BASE OF THE THUMB

➤ Check at the base of the thumb for sore spots or tenderness (Figure 14.63). Slowly rotate the thumb and move it toward or away from the palm until you find a position where the tenderness subsides. Then gently grasp the thumb and compress through the joints toward the base of the thumb and wrist and wait for ten to thirty seconds (Figures 14.64 and 14.65).

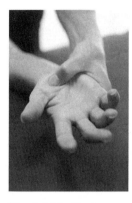 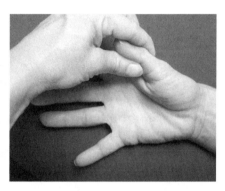 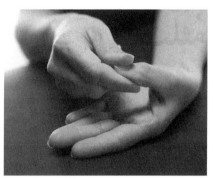

Fig. 14.63. Find tender point at base of thumb

Fig. 14.64. Rotate thumb and compress toward the base of the thumb

Fig. 14.65. Rotate thumb and compress toward the joint

※※※

CHAPTER 15

Neck

The neck can be thought of as the "control tower," as it creates the bridge between the brain and the rest of the body. Often the neck becomes tight and tense in response to our attempts to have more control over our lives. When we find ourselves overwhelmed by circumstances or situations, we might expend even greater effort to regain a sense of control, only to find our neck tight, tense, and aching from the effort.

If you are feeling overwhelmed, take a break—check in with your neck and the rest of your body, assess for comfort, recognize what is a realistic expectation of your capacity, and reassess your priorities.

Or better yet, release your neck before overwhelm sets in.

Anatomy

The neck is made up of seven cervical (neck) vertebrae extending from the base of the skull to the top of the shoulders where the thoracic spine begins. Optimally, these vertebrae form a slight anterior (forward) curve (Figure 15.1). Groups of large and small muscles provide flexibility and resilience within the neck and balanced support for the head. The movement of the neck allows for flexion (forward curling), extension (arching back), rotation (side-to-side "no" gesture), and lateral bending (ear toward shoulder) movements.

A head weighs around eleven pounds, and any cervical misalignment can cause the neck muscles to tighten in an attempt to balance the head. By releasing tension in the neck, functional alignment can be restored and supported, and range of motion and circulation enhanced.

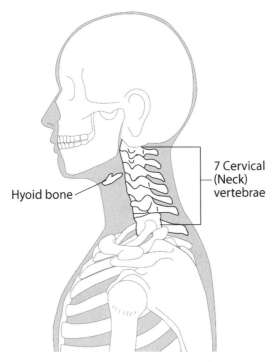

Fig. 15.1. Anatomy of the neck

General Positioning to Release the Neck

➤ To ease the neck, we are looking for a position of release and relaxation that most closely approximates the way the body is already holding itself in tension. By shortening the position of the tight muscles we offer an opportunity for release. For example, if the front of the neck is tight and sore on the right, the head may be drawn forward and rotated slightly to the right. To release this, support the back of the neck and head on a pillow so that the chin is closer to the chest. Slowly rotate the chin slightly to the right to aid in slackening the tense tissue (Figure 15.2).

For tender points along the sides of the neck, a combination move including rotation and side-bending that slackens the area around the point may be all that is necessary to soften and release the area of tension (Figure 15.3).

By moving very slowly in your exploration, you can fine-tune the positioning around tender points and create maximum softening around the tight or sore area. When a point loses its tenderness, you have reached an optimum position. You may notice softening to the touch or a slight pulsation as circulation returns to the area.

If you have multiple tender or tension points in the neck, just address each one individually, starting with the ones in the middle and then working the lower ones and finishing with the upper points. Also remember the importance of releasing the neighborhood points of the 1st rib and shoulders.

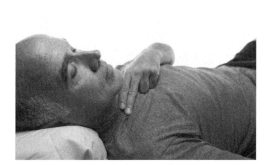

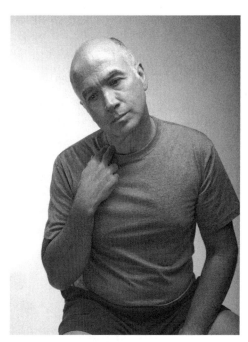

Figs. 15.2 and 15.3. Rotate and side-bend head toward tender point

General Releases Using Range-of-Motion Preferences

As you check for rotational and lateral bending preferences, it is important to move very slowly. This gives the nervous system an opportunity to release and recalibrate, and you have the opportunity to notice and affirm your comfort. If you move too quickly, there is a tendency to miss the optimal position for release.

Each of these releases may be done sitting, standing, or lying down. In cases of acute tension or pain, do the exercises lying on your back to relieve the neck of bearing the weight of the head and to offer greater support for the neck. If you are lying down, initiate the rotation movement from the back of the head where it is resting on the bed or floor. Allow the head to roll slowly from side to side, sensing the contact between the back of the head and the surface you're lying on.

ROLLING THE HEAD (ROTATING THE NECK)

➤ Lie on your back, and sensing the contact that your head makes with the bed or floor, slowly roll your head to the right and then back to center, and then slowly to the left and return to center. Note the direction of greater comfort and easier movement (Figures 15.4 to 15.6).

Rotate to the direction of greater comfort, stay there for ten to thirty seconds, and then return to center.

Recheck for increased range and comfort in the opposite direction.

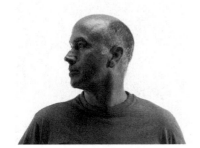
Fig. 15.4. Rotate neck to the right

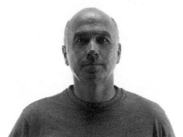
Fig. 15.5. Rotate back to center

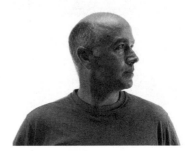
Fig. 15.6. Rotate neck to the left

DROPPING THE EAR (SIDE-BENDING THE NECK)

➤ Slowly allow your ear to fall sideways toward your shoulder. Notice any resistance or discomfort in the movement. Bring your head back to center and allow the other ear to fall laterally toward that shoulder. Notice to which side the neck bends more comfortably and easily (Figures 15.7 to 15.9).

Now move to that exact place of ease. You may support the neck with your hand in this place for ten to thirty seconds, allowing the tension to relax.

Return to center and recheck for more balanced range of motion and increased comfort.

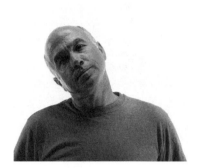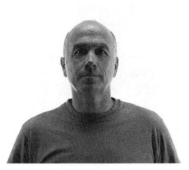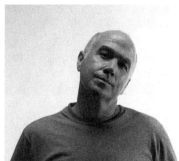

Figs. 15.7 to 15.9. Drop ear to shoulder

NOSE CIRCLES *,,,*

➤ Sitting or standing, slowly and gently let your nose fall toward your chest. From this position gently roll the nose over toward the shoulder, then up, slowly drawing your nose in a circle toward the ceiling, then down toward the other shoulder, and finally back down toward your chest (Figures 15.10 to 15.18).

As you draw this circle with your nose, note the places where movement feels restricted or uncomfortable. Many times, movement will feel restricted on one side of the circle, but the opposite side feels more relaxed or flexible. Gently move your nose to this place where the neck feels most at ease. Rest in this comfortable position for ten to thirty seconds (Figures 15.19 and 15.20).

Then slowly draw your nose circle again to see if there has been any change or release.

Be sure to draw nose circles in both directions.

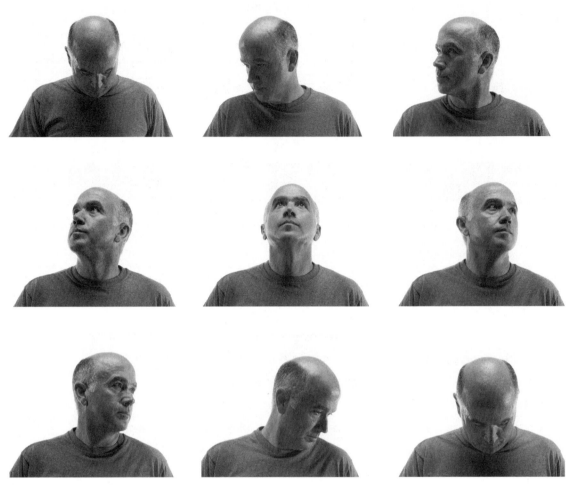

Figs. 15.10 to 15.18. Nose Circles to check for areas of tension

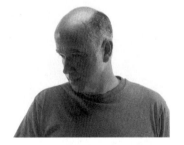

Fig. 15.19. Place of discomfort

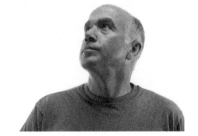

Fig. 15.20. Release position at opposite side of circle from discomfort or tension

ANOTHER PLACE OF COMFORT ON THE NOSE CIRCLE ,,,,,,,,,,,,,,,,,,,,,,,,,,,,,,,,,,,,,,,

➤ While making your nose circle, if you come across restriction or discomfort, go back just before the restriction and notice where there is a place of comfort. Rest your neck in that comfortable position for ten to thirty seconds. Then recheck to see if there is more freedom of movement in the restricted part (Figures 15.21 and 15.22).

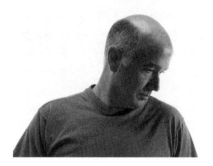

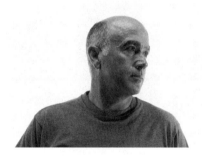

Fig. 15.21. Position of discomfort

Fig. 15.22. Position of release (just before place of discomfort or tension)

BACK-OF-NECK TENSION ,,,

➤ If you feel tension or tender points at the back of the neck, lightly place your finger on the tension point to monitor. Extend your chin up toward the ceiling until you feel a softening at the tissue under your monitoring finger (Figures 15.23 and 15.24).

Relax the neck muscles and remain in this position for thirty to sixty seconds. If you are doing this exercise while lying down, you can support your neck in this extended position with a pillow for greater relaxation.

You can use this position to release the 1st cervical vertebra where it connects to the base of the skull. Also try releasing the base of the skull with the Tennis Ball release (under "General Releases for the Head and Face" in Chapter 16).

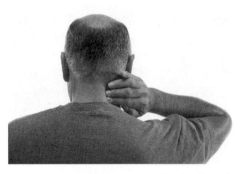

Fig. 15.23. Find tension at back of neck

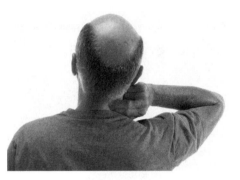

Fig. 15.24. Release position for back-of-neck tension

SIDES OF THE NECK

➤ If you feel tension or tender points at the side of the neck, place your middle finger on the point of tension as a monitor. Slowly and gently rotate and side-bend toward the side of the tension until the point softens or begins to pulsate (Figures 15.25 and 15.26).

Remain in this position for ten to thirty seconds. You may hold any of these positions longer if it allows for deeper relaxation of tension.

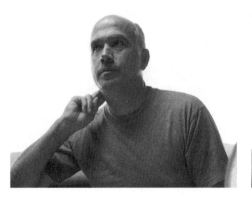

Fig. 15.25. Find tenderness on side of neck

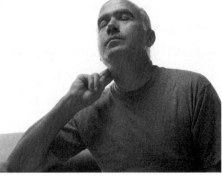

Fig. 15.26. Release position for tender points on side of neck

LOWER NECK ///

➤ If there is a tender point at the base of the neck where it meets the shoulder, set up the release position by first rotating the head away from the sore point (Figure 15.27). Next, slowly rotate the head back toward center (midline). Stop anywhere along that path when you notice a softening at the point. Hold the release position for ten to twenty seconds (Figure 15.28).

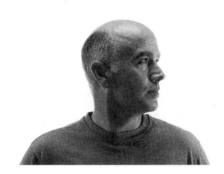

Fig. 15.27. Rotate head away from tender point at base of neck

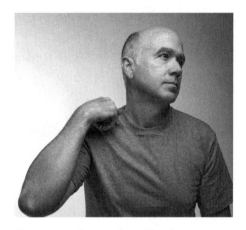

Fig. 15.28. Rotate head back to midline, stopping when point softens

FRONT OF THE NECK ///

➤ If you sense tension, contraction, or tender points at the front of your neck, bend your head forward into flexion and add a slight side bend and rotation to create a softening around the tender point until it begins to pulsate or soften. Stay in this comfortable position for ten to thirty seconds.

If you are trying this positioning while lying on your back, prop the head into flexion with a pillow (Figure 15.29).

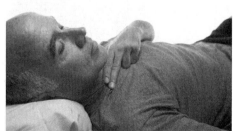

Fig. 15.29. Front of the neck release position

TREATING WHIPLASH //

In a whiplash injury, the neck is moved very quickly in one direction and then is whipped back in the opposite direction. Small muscles between the vertebrae (intrinsic muscles) tighten to prevent injury to the discs and spinal cord. Sometimes after the injury, though, these small muscles are still holding on for dear life and impede the natural return to flexibility.

The releases for whiplash injuries tend to be the *opposite* of those that are normally used for tension patterns in the neck. For example, in a whiplash injury, if the right side of the neck feels tight and tense, you may need to curve (rotate and side-bend) toward the left to get a release (Figures 15.30 and 15.31). If the tension is in the back of the neck, flattening the natural anterior cervical curve, then you may need to flex the head toward the chest to get the neck to release.

Remember to slowly explore for the most comfortable position. Monitor the point for softening and relaxation of the tissues. Moving very slowly and gently keeps you from activating any reactive defensive patterns that could interfere with the release.

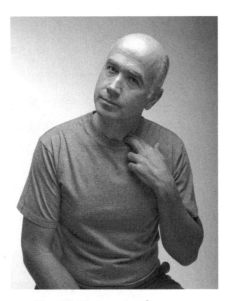

Fig. 15.30. Locate place
of whiplash tension

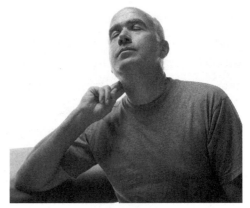

Fig. 15.31. Release point on the
opposite side of whiplash tension

RELEASING TRAUMA IN THE NECK *,,*

Defensive patterns that can be held within the tiny intrinsic muscles of the neck sometimes require even more subtle treatment. After my motorcycle accident, my neck was hypersensitive to any sudden movement. I was able to desensitize it with a combination of subtle movement and meditation.

Use this exercise if your neck is very sensitive or reactive. Practice it on days when you feel like relaxing and have some uninterrupted time for yourself.

➤ Begin by lying on your back, calming your mind, and resting quietly for a few minutes. Very slowly, allow your neck to rotate only about an eighth to a quarter of an inch to one side. Then rest for a few minutes, allowing your whole self to totally relax and your mind to drift.

When you have finished your daydream, allow your neck to move an eighth to a quarter of an inch further. Once again, completely relax your whole body and let the mind empty. The idea is to allow the neck and any tension reflexes to release at each angle within a neck rotation (Figures 15.32 to 15.34).

To fully release the trauma pattern in the neck may require more than one self-care session. Allow yourself all the time you need for each release.

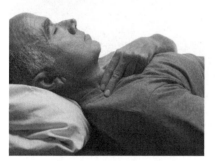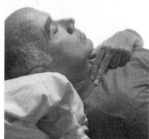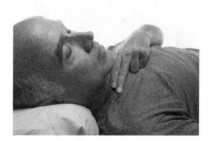

Figs. 15.32 to 15.34. Incremental rotational release of neck trauma

PAINTBRUSH MOVEMENT EXERCISE FOR THE NECK *,,*

Here is another exercise from Gerda Alexander's Eutony[1] class that is so effective in releasing neck tension. You may feel a bit silly or self-conscious at first, but the results will get your attention.

➤ Standing or sitting comfortably, imagine that you have a paintbrush or a marker in your ear. Slowly initiate comfortable movements as if you were painting in the air with your ear.

Allow the rest of your body to follow the movements initiated by your ear. Staying in your comfort range with your body following the ear's lead, paint your masterpiece in the air for two to three minutes (Figures 15.35 to 15.43).

Then compare your sense of one side of the neck with the other. Switch your imaginary paintbrush to the other ear and repeat the process.

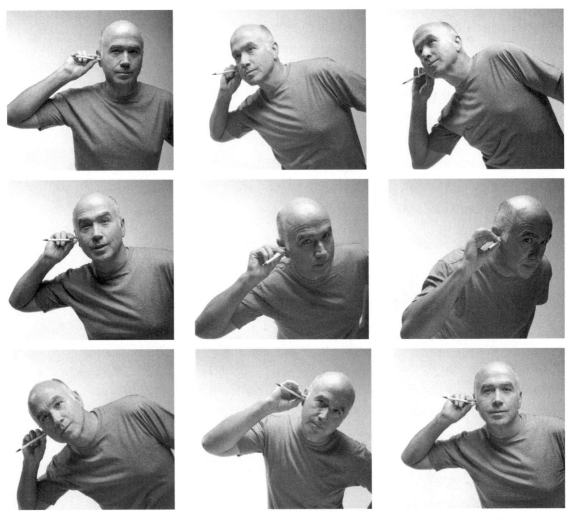

Figs. 15.35 to 15.43. Drawing with an imaginary paintbrush
or pen in the ear to release neck tension

※※※

CHAPTER 16

Head, Face, Eyes, Ears, and Jaw

Sometimes we feel helpless when tension or pain occurs in the head. Introducing very gentle movements to the face, nose, ears, and head helps us notice which specific movements release tension, create comfort, and initiate relaxation for ourselves.

Head pain can be the result of tension and stress in other parts of the body. To effectively reduce recurring head pain, we need to release tension patterns in the neck, shoulders, 1st rib, and spine as well.

General Releases for the Head and Face

RELEASING TENSION

➤ Place your fingertips on your face or head. Slowly and gently assess the preferred direction of skin movement, allowing the fingertips to follow the movement preferences of the skin tissue.

The sensations may seem subtle, but essentially you follow the tissue in one direction until movement seems to stop, and then you make a right turn or left turn to see which direction is preferred. Continue to follow the tissue until the next place it stops, then turn again in the direction of preference. Continue following the skin preferences until you feel relaxed or until the skin and tissue seem to move in all directions with ease (Figures 16.1 to 16.4).

You can work with the tiny muscles in the face and jaw in the same way. Just let the fingers follow the sensed movement preferences.

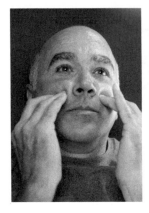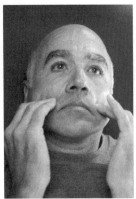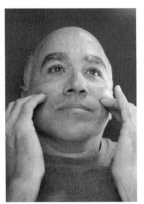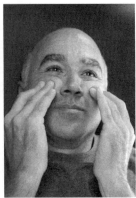

Figs. 16.1 to 16.4. Explore movement preference to relax the face

RELEASING THE BASE OF THE SKULL (TENNIS BALL RELEASE)〟〟〟〟〟〟〟〟〟〟〟

Many times a headache is caused by tension at the top of the neck where it meets the base of the skull.

➤ Put two tennis balls into a sock and tie a knot at the end. Lie down and place the tennis balls under the base of your head where it meets the neck. Let your head rest on the tennis balls (Figures 16.5 to 16.7). An eye pillow (a small rectangular pillow filled with flax seeds or lavender) placed over the eyes is also useful.

Imagine and allow your eyes to drop back in their sockets toward the tennis balls. Stay quiet and rest in this position for five to ten minutes.

It may be helpful to first release the 1st rib, Shoulder Point 8, and the sides and back of the neck.

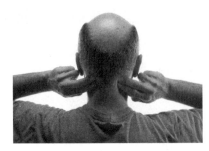

Fig. 16.5. Check for tension at base of skull and top of neck

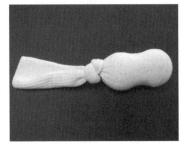

Fig. 16.6. Two tennis balls in a sock

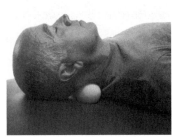

Fig. 16.7. Head rests on tennis balls to release base of skull

RELEASING THE HEAD BY RELEASING THE BRIDGE OF THE NOSE ,,,,,,,,,,,,,,,,,,

Years ago Arthur Pauls talked about a practitioner in Europe who claimed to be able to release any part of the body just by making subtle movements on the bridge of the nose. I remember my skepticism and dismissal of the whole story as one of Arthur's tall tales.

Yet less than a month later, I awoke in the middle of the night to find my fingers on the bridge of my nose making tiny subtle adjustments and sensing these movements releasing the tension and pain in my head. I could feel each of the various positions releasing different areas of my head. It was incredibly effective.

Try it for yourself and see.

➤ Lightly rest your thumb and forefinger on either side of the bridge of your nose. Experiment with applying very slight amounts of pressure in different directions along the sides of the nose.

As you make the tiny, subtle movements, try to get a sense of which area of the head is affected by each position and direction (Figures 16.8 to 16.11).

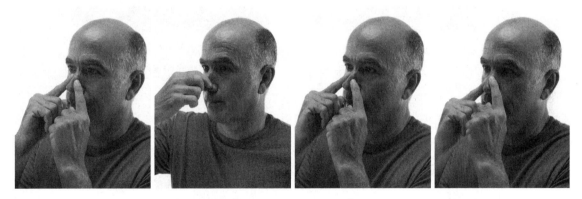

Figs. 16.8 to 16.11. Explore movement preferences
of the nose to release head tension

ANOTHER NOSE RELEASE

➤ Lightly rest your thumb and forefinger on either side of the cartilage of your nose. Very, very slowly move the nose to one side and then the other. Hold in the position that feels most comfortable to you for ten to thirty seconds and release.

Next, gently push the bridge of the nose up toward the forehead and then down toward the chin. Hold in the position that feels best to you for ten to thirty seconds and release (Figures 16.12 and 16.13).

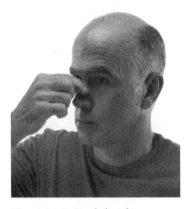

Fig. 16.12. Push bridge
of nose up (toward forehead)

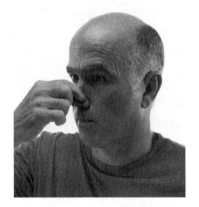

Fig. 16.13. Push bridge of
nose down (toward chin)

NOSE AND CHEEK RELEASE

Perhaps you've heard the expression, "Don't get your nose pushed out of shape." If you haven't heeded that advice, here's a release just for that. Remember, if your nose is curved one way, just take it a little bit further in the same direction and then it can self-correct.

The pressure in this exercise is not as subtle as in the last two.

➤ Move the cartilage of your nose to one side, then to the other. Hold it to the side that feels more comfortable.

With your other hand, stroke with your finger down the opposite side of the nose and cheek (Figures 16.14 to 16.16).

Then switch and repeat on the other side.

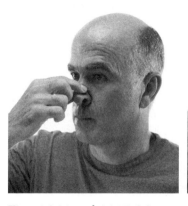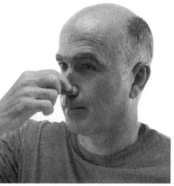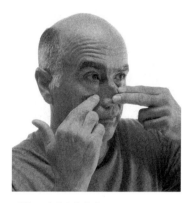

Figs. 16.14 and 16.15. Move nose to one side and the other

Fig. 16.16. Move nose to comfortable side and rub down side of cheek

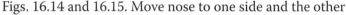

Eyes

Sometimes referred to as "the windows of the soul," our eyes communicate much about our overall health. In an introductory class in iridology, I studied the correlation between the markings within the iris and the physical health of the body. I was most fascinated by observing the eye through a lighted magnifier and learning to read the map of the eyes. Seeing the eye like a floating world was an awe-inspiring experience.

Just as all the tissues and structures of the body need adequate circulation to maintain healthy functioning, so do our eyes. Their health is negatively impacted by tension in the muscles behind the eyes and by poor circulation that reduces the amount of nutrients the eyes receive.

You may have noticed that when you are feeling relaxed and well-rested, you actually see better.

General Releases

These exercises reduce tension in the muscles that support the eyeball, so that they help relax the eyes, release eyestrain, and increase circulation to the eyes, allowing nutrients to better reach the tissues.

➤ Contact the closed eyelids with a very light touch. Always stay with your comfort. You will get much better results by working gently, slowly, and lightly.

EYE TAPPING

Lightly place the tip of your middle finger on the closed eyelid. Using the fingernail of the index finger of the opposite hand, tap *very gently* on the fingernail of the finger resting on the closed eyelid (Figure 16.17).

This tapping sets up a vibration that relaxes the muscles behind the eyes and increases circulation to the muscles and nerves of the eyes.

You may move the contact finger to different positions and continue tapping to release the various areas of the eye.

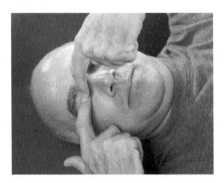

Fig. 16.17. Gentle tapping on finger to release eye tension

EYE BALANCING

➤ Carefully place the fingertips of your middle fingers on one closed eyelid, one at each corner of the eye. Very gently initiate a movement to lightly push the eyeball to one side and then to the other (Figures 16.18 and 16.19).

Notice any restriction to movement and note which position or direction feels most comfortable. Hold in the position of comfort for three to five seconds. If there is no preference, hold to the side that moves most easily.

Then release and recheck by moving the eyeball back and forth and noting any changes.

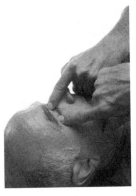

Fig. 16.18. Gently rock eyeball medial (toward nose)

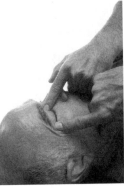

Fig. 16.19. Gently rock eyeball lateral (toward ear)

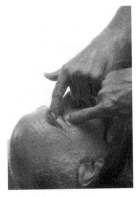

Fig. 16.20. Gently rock eyeball up (toward top of head)

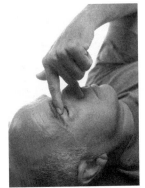

Fig. 16.21. Gently rock eyeball down (toward feet)

Also check for top-to-bottom and diagonal movement preferences of the eyeball (Figures 16.20 to 16.25). Hold in each position of preference for three to five seconds. Then release and recheck for greater movement.

You may finish with the eye tapping exercise above.

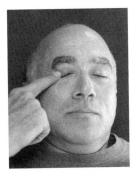

Fig. 16.22. Gently rock eyeball diagonally (up and in)

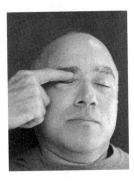

Fig. 16.23. Gently rock eyeball diagonally (down and out)

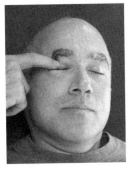

Fig. 16.24. Gently rock eyeball diagonally (down and in)

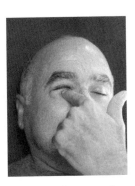

Fig. 16.25. Gently rock eyeball diagonally (out and up)

Ears

EAR MASSAGE

Shaped like the fetus from which we all developed, the ears hold reflexes to all the parts of the body. A gentle ear massage can release tension in the head, neck, and much of the rest of the body.

➤ Gently massage your ears with your fingertips and thumb. Use slow circular movements beginning at the tops and work down the sides to the lobes. Gently squeeze the skin between your fingers and thumb, noting how much pressure feels comfortable. Repeat any movements that feel good and help you to relax (Figures 16.26 and 16.27).

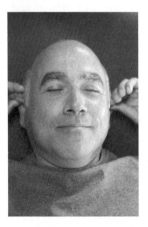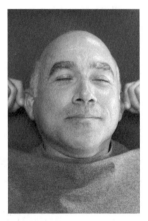

Figs. 16.26 and 16.27. Ear massage

EAR PULLS

➤ Very gently pull your ears out and away from your head. Sense the stretch of the skin behind the ears where they meet the head. Can you sense a subtle "recoil" of the stretched tissue naturally pulling the ears back toward the head? That's the body's signal to you to release the pull (Figure 16.28).

Compare your two sides. Does one side seem tighter than the other? Can you play with the tension, pulling on one ear and feeling any effect on the other side? Can you sense the membrane pull through the head, connecting the movement between the ears? If not, just imagine the connection and play with the gentle pull back and forth until both sides let go of any tension or until both sides come into balance.

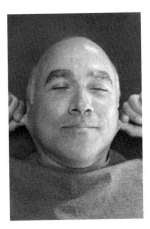

Fig. 16.28. Gentle ear pulls

❦❦❦

Jaw: General Releases

In the ancient Chinese *Book of Changes,* the *I Ching,* there is a reference to the mouth in regard to providing nourishment. The teaching image states, "The superior man is careful of his words and temperate in his eating and drinking."[1] The muscles of the jaw allow us to both chew our food and speak the thoughts of our mind and heart.

The position of the jaw can serve as an expression of attitude or emotion. Many of us hold tension in our jaw, and we discover it tight and clenched at night as our unconscious tries to grind and chew through all the issues we didn't resolve during the day. You may have felt your own jaw quiver before tears start to flow, or noticed a child jut out his jaw and protrude the lower lip in an expression of disappointment.

The jaw and the pelvis reflex to each other.[2] Just as the pelvis is the bowl-shaped floor of the torso, the jaw creates the structural floor of the mouth. So the release positions and movement exercises for the pelvis and low back may benefit the jaw as well.

PELVIC RELEASE FOR THE JAW ,,,

This exercise came to me while teaching a class. When an insistent student wanted me to demonstrate a jaw release, I decided to try an exploratory approach. I watched the person slowly open and close his jaw. I noted the places of hesitation in the movement and where the jaw jagged to the right or left, which revealed an unevenness of the muscle use patterns on either side of the jaw. Intuitively, I wondered if a quick release of the pelvis would reflex to the jaw. I was just as surprised as everyone else in the class when this simple release worked so quickly. It has become a favorite self-care exercise because it is so easy and effective.

➤ Begin this exercise by lying on your back with your knees raised and feet resting on the floor. Very, very slowly open your mouth, noting any areas where the jaw feels tight or seems to slide or pull to one side or the other. Then very slowly close your mouth, noting any discomfort or tension as you close.

Repeat the opening and closing, this time stopping at the first place that you notice any deviation or tension. Hold your mouth open at this place and let your knees fall to one side. It doesn't matter to which side—you may let them fall to the right or to the left, or one leg to each side (Figures 16.29 and 16.30).

Rest the legs in the fallen position with the mouth open for three to five seconds, no longer. Then, as you slowly let the legs slide down fully extended to the floor, slowly close your mouth (Figures 16.31 to 16.33).

Slowly open your mouth again and recheck for any release or change in the tension pattern.

*You may repeat this exercise for **only one** more tension spot in the jaw. It is best to limit this exercise to two repetitions per self-care session in order to optimize the integration of the new pattern and not fatigue the reflex.*

Fig. 16.29. Slowly open the mouth

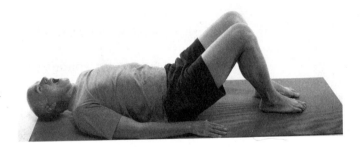

Fig. 16.30. Let legs drop to either side (keep mouth open)

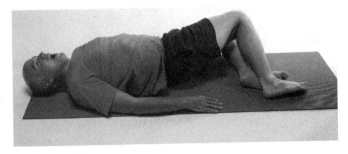

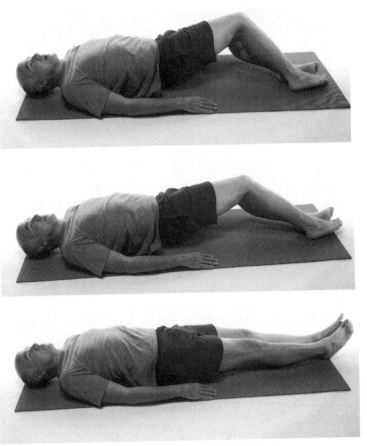

Figs. 16.31 to 16.33. Slowly extend the legs and let the mouth close

RELEASING THE MUSCLES OF THE JAW

➤ Place the palms of your hands on the side of your face with your fingers pointing up. Gently push your cheeks and jaw muscles up toward your temples with your palms. Hold for ten to twenty seconds, then release and gently and slowly pull down on the cheeks (Figures 16.34 and 16.35).

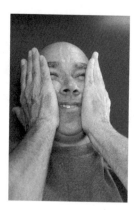
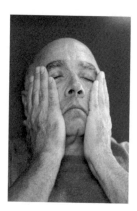

Figs. 16.34 and 16.35. Release the muscles of the jaw

※※※

IV. Special Conditions

✲ ✲ ✲

CHAPTER 17

Sciatica

Sciatica is an irritating, achy nerve pain in the buttocks that can radiate down the leg. It can result from tension in the low back (lumbar spine region) or from a rotated hip bone (ilium) that causes tightness at the sacroiliac joint. An injury or inefficient postural pattern can cause an imbalance in the muscles of the sacroiliac joint, creating pressure on the sciatic nerve (Figure 17.1).

An imbalance of the muscles in the hips and buttocks causing sciatic pain can be the result of a postural habit such as sitting with your wallet in your back pocket. If one hip is always sitting a bit higher than the other, then the hip muscles on either side of the sacrum are not working evenly. If the wallet is the culprit then you have two choices for relief. Either remove the wallet or, as I would tell my clients, wait until you have spent all your money on practitioners in vain attempts to feel better. Just as we saw with the contractor who needed to wear his tool belt reversed for half the day, the body cannot learn to hold a more balanced structure if it continues to work in an imbalanced way.

Be sure to use the release positions and movement exercises for the rotated ilium, sacrum, and lumbar region to restore balance to the sciatic neighborhoods.

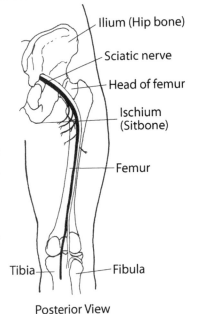

Fig. 17.1. Sciatic nerve. Courtesy of *Illustrated Essentials of Musculoskeletal Anatomy,* 4th Edition, by Sieg and Adams (Gainesville, FL: Megabooks, Inc., 1992), www.muscleanatomybook.com.

Ilium (Hip bone)

Sciatic nerve

Head of femur

Ischium (Sitbone)

Femur

Tibia

Fibula

Posterior View

Try the following self-care techniques at the first sign of sciatic discomfort:

- Release the low back and the 5th lumbar specifically (Chapter 2)
- Check and release rotated ilium (hip bone) (Chapter 3)
- Use the Lazy Dog release position (Chapter 3)
- Knee releases (Chapter 6)

Movement Exercises to Relieve Sciatic Discomfort

The following two exercises are specific and effective for relieving sciatic pain and discomfort in the moment and can be used anytime.

SCIATIC CURTSY

➤ Stand where you can hold on to a support. Shift your weight off the painful (affected) leg and cross it over the other leg, with the toes of the affected leg just touching down for balance. Curtsy from the knees. Bend and straighten several times (Figures 17.2 and 17.3).

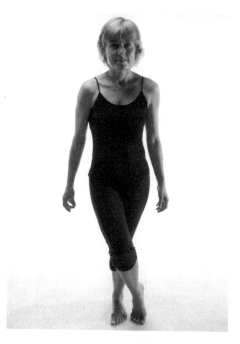 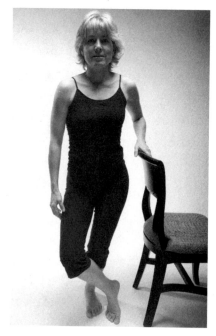

Figs. 17.2 and 17.3. Sciatic Curtsy

SCIATIC SLIDE //

➤ Stand with the affected foot (the one on the painful side) forward about the length of a natural step and bend your knees slightly. Keeping your knees bent, your feet flat on the floor, and your hips level, shift your weight forward over your front foot by sliding your hips forward and then slide them back, shifting your weight backward over your rear foot (Figures 17.4 and 17.5).

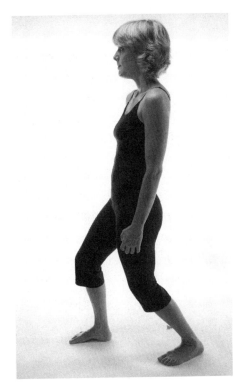

Fig. 17.4. Sciatic Slide forward

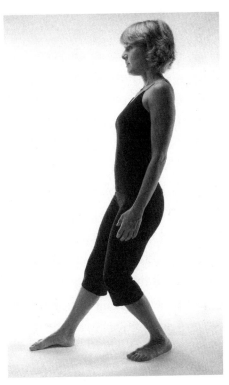

Fig. 17.5. Sciatic Slide back

Movement Exercises to Maintain Flexibility in the Sacroiliac Joint

Walking is one of the most useful activities for pain in the sacrum and sacroiliac region. Instead of going to bed to rest when you feel discomfort or tension in this area, take a short walk. Walking can be a very effective way to remind the body of its natural capacity to return balance to this area. More information on walking can be found in Chapter 9.

Movement exercises important for opening and maintaining flexibility in the sacroiliac joint are repeated here (from the section on the Sacrum).

SUPINE KICKING FOR SCIATICA ,,,

This movement exercise is good for sciatica and releases tension all along the spine. It is especially good for those who have been bedridden with sciatica, as it reminds the sacroiliac joint of its ability to move without having to bear weight.

➤ Lying on your back, bend your left knee so you rest your left foot on the floor. The right leg is still flat (extended) on the floor. Now slide the heel of the right (extended) leg toward your buttocks, bending your right knee up toward the ceiling. At the same time, let the heel of the left leg slide down so the leg flops down to an extended position on the floor. Repeat the heel sliding movement, flopping one leg down as you simultaneously raise the opposite knee (Figures 17.6 to 17.8).

You can increase the pace to feel like you are having a mini-tantrum. Just make sure that the accent of the movement is on the flop, not the lift. If this exercise bothers your knees, place a small pillow under your knees for support during the flopping.

Do this one for a minute or two. Or stop when you are tired. Just let each leg end up by flopping on the floor or pillow (if you have used one under your knees).

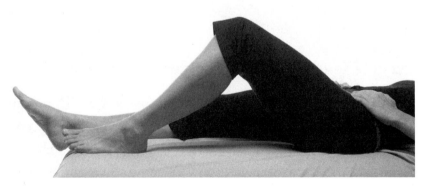

Fig. 17.6. Slide left heel up as right leg slides down

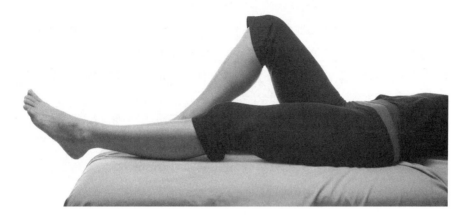

Fig. 17.7. Slide right heel up as left leg slides down

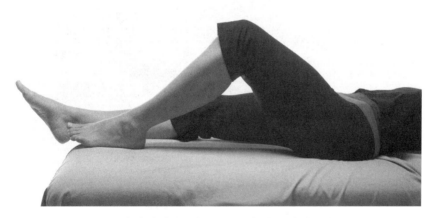

Fig. 17.8. Slide left heel up as right leg slides down

TEENAGE TELEPHONE TALK //

➤ Lying on your abdomen (prone), bend your knees so your feet are up in the air. Slowly draw circles in the air with your feet, noting where in the circle there is more ease and comfort. You may pause and rest in the comfortable positions for a few moments (Figure 17.9).

This exercise is named "Teenage Telephone Talk" because it captures the mood of a relaxed teen, unconsciously self-balancing the pelvis while chatting on the phone. You can also think of it as a slow leg spin.

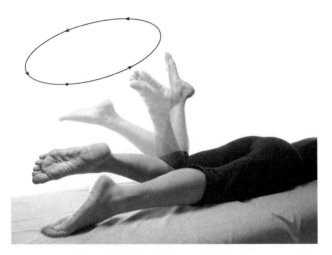

Fig. 17.9. Teenage Telephone Talk (Slow Leg Spin)

SCISSORS //

➤ Lying on your abdomen (prone), bend your knees so your feet are up in the air. Let the feet swing out to the sides and then toward each other, crossing the midline like scissors. Bring your attention to your sacroiliac joints as you do these movements. Keep your movements slow and easy—this is not an aerobic workout (Figure 17.10 to 17.12).

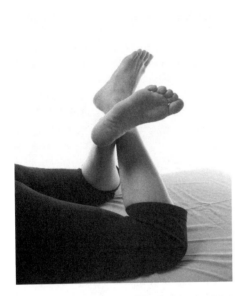
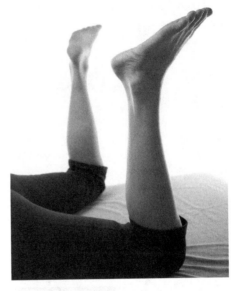
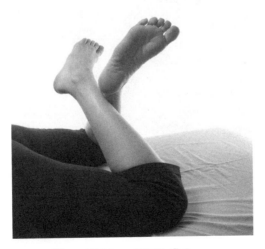

Figs. 17.10 to 17.12. Scissors

FOOT AND LEG RUB

This exercise increases flexibility in the sacroiliac joint.

➤ Lie on your abdomen with your knees bent and your feet in the air.

Rub your feet against each other, touching all the surfaces together. Remember to include the tops and sides of the feet. Notice if one foot is more active in the movement than the other, and balance the movement action between the feet (Figures 17.13 to 17.15).

Then rub down the inside of each leg with the opposing foot (Figures 17.16 to 17.18).

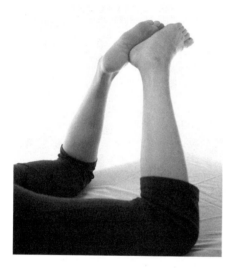
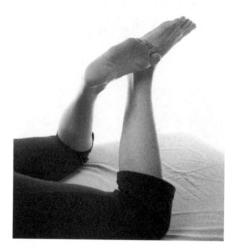
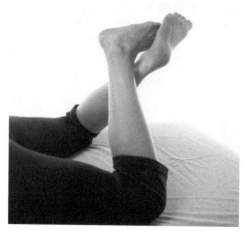

Figs. 17.13 to 17.15. Foot Rub for sacroiliac joint flexibility

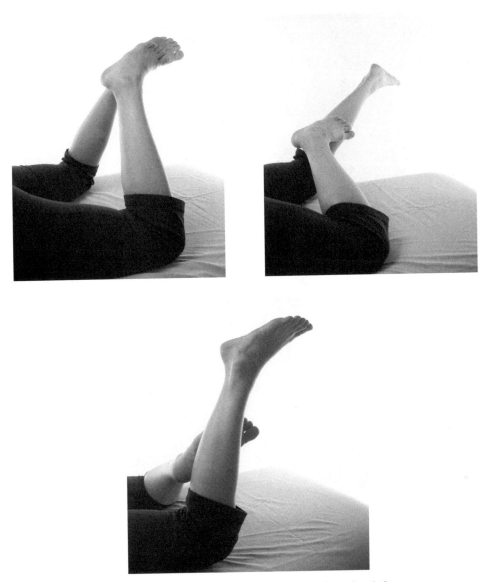

Figs. 17.16 to 17.18. Leg Rub for sacroiliac flexibility

※※※

CHAPTER 18

Bunions

Arthur Pauls taught that this technique if repeated nightly corrects bunions, and many students with bunions have confirmed this with their own experience. According to Pauls, bunions get worse when the ligament along the outside of the big toe slips off its track, allowing the big toe joint to expand out to the side of the foot. It is important to first release the joint at the bunion and then to reeducate the big toe to resume its natural positioning. Repeating this release exercise nightly is an essential part of the reeducation process. Once the big toe gradually recovers and sustains its alignment, the ligament can then be manipulated back to its original supportive position.

BUNION RELEASE

➤ Slightly exaggerate the position of the big toe and bunion by rotating and moving the big toe closer to the other toes. In this position compress the big toe along the line of the bone straight back toward the bunion. Fine-tune the position for comfort. Hold the position with compression toward the joint for ten to thirty seconds and release. Then gently pull the big toe outward toward an aligned position (Figures 18.1 and 18.2).

Place a soft cotton cloth between the big toe and the second toe to help hold the alignment. Then place a band for bunions (available at your pharmacy) across the long foot bones (metatarsals) that connect to the toes. This will hold the foot in alignment while you sleep.

I have also seen all-in-one bunion devices advertised at www.skymall.com and www.footsmart.com. These have both parts combined and would work well to reeducate alignment of the big toe after you have completed the release.

Repeat this release nightly to improve and reeducate the big toe toward alignment.

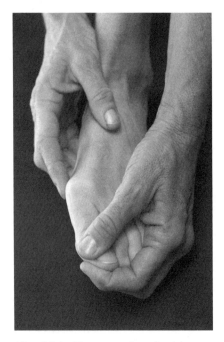

Fig. 18.1. Compressing the big toe toward bunion

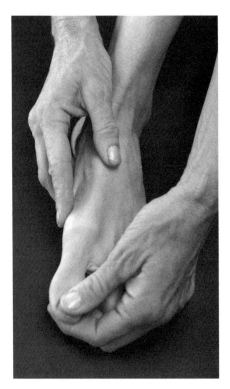

Fig. 18.2. Pulling the big toe after compression release

※※※

CHAPTER 19

Scoliosis

What Is It?

When the spine develops sideways (lateral) curves or fixated rotational patterns, the condition is called scoliosis. In most cases, the exact cause is unknown. Many times scoliosis runs in families. It may have genetic origins or arise from imitating postural patterns during early childhood.

A raised shoulder, usually the right, a higher hip, a protruding shoulder blade, or a rounded area in the upper or lower back can be indicative of scoliosis (Figures 19.1 to 19.3). Most cases are mild, but in a small percentage of cases the effects may be more complicated and can cause heart and lung problems. While not always painful, common complaints associated with scoliosis include back pain, arm and shoulder tension and pain, discrepancy in leg length, and endocrine or nervous system imbalances. Pain and discomfort can vary from mild soreness to a sensation of muscle fatigue with achy numbness or tingling. The feeling of being out of alignment can cause irritation, frustration, and increased tension.

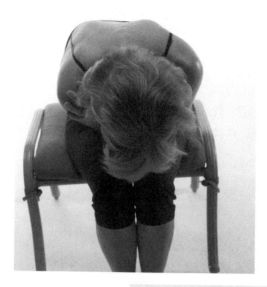

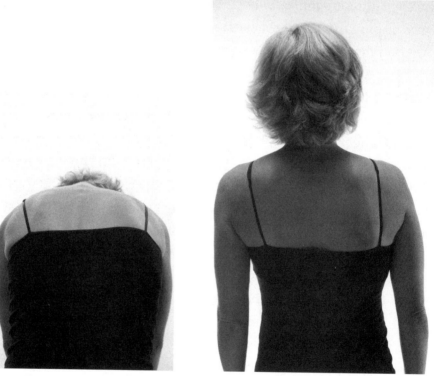

Figs. 19.1 to 19.3. Positions in which to view scoliosis—notice the rotation (twist) in rib cage and shoulder and the protrusion of the right shoulder blade. Sometimes with scoliosis the spine will appear to have an "S" curve when the person bends forward.

Suggested Positional Release and Exercise Sequence for Addressing Scoliosis

From an Ortho-Bionomy perspective, scoliosis is addressed in three ways: release holding patterns in the pelvis, spine, and rib cage; reestablish balanced range of movement in the pelvis, spine, and rib cage; and reeducate the spinal curves. Awareness exercises help you to attune to the area, assess your preferences, and recognize "glitches" and imbalances in your movement patterns. The release positions relax tension and fixated muscular holding patterns. Gentle movement exercises reeducate the spinal muscles to an increased range of movement and a more balanced sense of dynamic alignment. Slow, exploratory movements with awareness allow the body to recognize a greater range of movement options, and to gradually reestablish more functionally balanced patterns of use.

Scoliosis affects different muscle groups in different people. For some it correlates with uneven use of pelvic and low-back muscles, while in others the major tension patterns seem to be in the rib cage, diaphragm, and spinal muscles. In most cases there is a habitual patterned way of moving that continues to strengthen the tight muscle patterns. It is as if there is a misunderstanding in the body regarding potential balanced movement so a patterned tension movement jumps in to compensate. Slowly and with awareness these patterned tensions can be released step by step and gently reeducated.

Below you will find a reference guide to some of the possible release positions and movement exercises useful for scoliosis, along with chapter numbers to find them in this book (utilize the Table of Contents for page number). Choose the ones that seem the best for releasing your particular tension patterns. The exercises replicated here with photos are the keys for reeducating the spine back to alignment and balanced posture. It is recommended that you go to the specific chapters for preparatory releases and a more thorough understanding of each exercise. Remember to give yourself time to approach the exercises slowly and with mindfulness.

The release positions and movement exercises combined with awareness help to relax the tension patterns so the spinal curves gradually become more balanced. Awareness of the sit bones and moving slowly in the "Finding the Midpoint" exercise helps the hips learn to move coherently so the muscles work evenly on both sides. The Disc Fluffer exercises combined with the rotation preference of the thoracic spine begin to free up movement potential in the upper-back area.

Once you are able to move the low back independently ("Finding the Midpoint") from the thoracic area (upper back), then you can begin to work toward a Balanced Sitting Posture. The exercises involved in Balanced Sitting Posture are the keys to unlock and reeducate the tiny muscle holdings of the spinal muscles and to retrain the spine to healthy curves. They consist of:

- Combining Disc Fluffer with Finding your Midpoint (Chapter 11).

- Combine Rotation and Side-Bend Preference to Create a Visually Straight Spine (in this chapter).

- Supporting the Natural Curves While You Sleep—a bedtime towel exercise to maintain flexibility and spinal curves (Chapter 11).

Begin with Awareness, Movement, and Releases for the Low Back and Pelvis

- Releases and isometric exercises as needed for the lumbar spine (to increase flexibility of the low back) are found in Chapter 2.

- Releases as needed for the ilium (hip) and sacrum (to balance hips and movement exercises to increase flexibility) are found in Chapter 3.

LOW BACK RELEASE POSITION WITH ABDOMINAL BREATHING (CHAPTER 2)

➤ Lie on your back on the floor. Bend your knees and rest your lower legs on a chair or couch. Your heels and lower legs will be resting at knee level or slightly above. Slowly move your knees, one at a time, slightly to the side or closer to your chest, exploring and adjusting until you find just the right position that feels most comfortable for your lower back (Figure 19.4).

While lying there comfortably, place your hands on your abdomen and inhale slowly and deeply. Your abdomen will rise as breath fills and inflates your lower lungs and then chest. Slowly exhale, and the abdomen will fall and soften. Imagine the air leaving gently and slowly through the lower back. Sense the abdomen rising with inhalation and softening at exhalation. Sense the breath moving through the low back during exhalation.

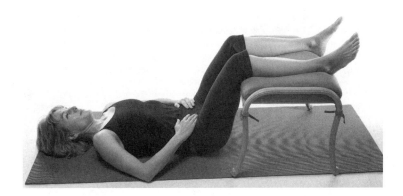

Fig. 19.4. Low Back Release Position with Abdominal Breathing

PELVIC CURL WITH BREATHING (CHAPTER 2)

➤ Lie on your back with knees bent and feet on the floor. Line up your knees and feet with your hips. Begin abdominal breathing—long, slow inhalations that allow your abdomen to rise—and imagine each exhalation exiting through your low back.

When you have established a relaxed rhythm with your breathing, during an exhalation gently push through your feet so there is more weight on your soles. Allow the push to transfer through the legs, gently rocking the pelvis and curling the pubic bone up toward the ceiling. As the pubic bone curls up, the low back will flatten toward the floor (Figure 19.6).

As you inhale, slowly release the weight from the feet and allow the abdomen to rise and the pelvis to passively rock back to neutral (Figure 19.5).

Continue the gentle push-through-feet to curl the pelvis upward during exhalation and to rock back to neutral during inhalation. Allow the abdominal muscles to remain relaxed throughout this exercise, as the breath moves in and out without pressure or forcing.

Movement with the breath adds relaxation and encourages slow, aware, and balanced movement in the lower back and pelvis. Slow, non-weight-bearing movement assists the body in letting go of patterned imbalanced movement.

If you have trouble syncing your breath with the movement, let go of the focus on the breath and just allow the movement. Refer to the "Press and Release" exercise in Chapter 2 for assistance.

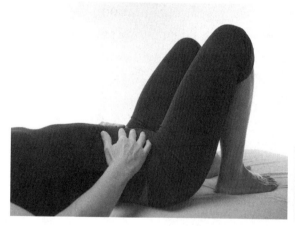

Fig. 19.5. Inhale, weight off feet

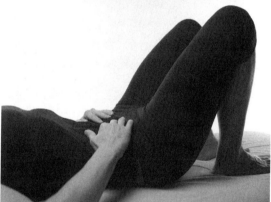

Fig. 19.6. Exhale, push on feet to curl pelvis

RELEASE POSITION FOR THE 5TH LUMBAR: DROPPED LEG (CHAPTER 2)*,,,,,,,*

This release is one of the most important in all cases of low back and pelvis tension. Refer to Chapter 2 for ways to assess the indicator point and alternative release positions.

➤ Lie on your abdomen (prone) on the bed with the affected side near the edge. Move your lower body to the edge and your upper body diagonally away, so that you can drop your leg off the side. Your bent knee is pointing to the floor, and your foot rests lightly on the floor (Figure 19.7). You want to give into gravity, feeling as much of a natural drop from the hip as is possible and comfortable. Do not try to support your weight from your low back, groin area, or dropped leg. Allow your entire body to relax into this position for a few minutes.

To come out of this release position, slide your other leg off the bed as well, so that you stand up by slowly putting weight onto both feet on the floor. The slide-off approach allows your back to maintain the release and prevents reestablishing the strain pattern. (If you try to lift your dropped leg back onto the bed, you may undo the release and reestablish the tension pattern.) Remember to move into and come out of these positions slowly so as to fine-tune the position and preserve the release (Figures 2.12 to 2.17 in Chapter 2).

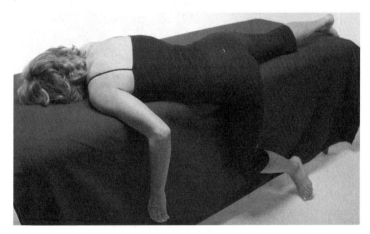

Fig. 19.7. 5th Lumbar Release Position—
a key release for the lower back

❆❆❆

Hip Releases from Chapter 3

These next two release positions help to unlock the muscle tension patterns in the hips that can create uneven leg length and unbalance the spine. See Chapter 3 for ways to assess hip (ilium) rotation; to perform releases for the sacrum and quadratus lumborum muscle; and to learn additional movement exercises to increase flexibility.

FROG POSITION TO RELEASE POSTERIOR HIP ROTATION (SHORTER LEG) (CHAPTER 3) ,,

➤ Lie on your abdomen and slowly bend your knee, bringing it out to the side of your body. This will rotate the hip a bit more posterior. We refer to this as the Frog position (Figure 19.8).

This release position and the next one help to unlock muscle tension patterns in the hips that can create uneven leg length and restrict the hips from rotating evenly.

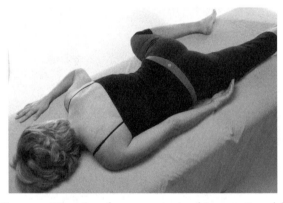

Fig. 19.8. Frog position to release posterior hip rotation (shorter leg)

RELEASE POSITION FOR ANTERIOR HIP ROTATION (LONGER LEG) (CHAPTER 3) ⫰⫰

➤ Stand at the corner at the end of a bed and rest your upper thigh and knee on the bed. Place your hands on the bed and support your upper body on your fully extended arms. Allow the front of the hip bone (ASIS) to drop slightly toward the bed. This will rotate the hip a bit more anterior. You may need to bend your standing knee a little.

Maintain this position, if comfortable for the hip, for ten to thirty seconds (Figure 19.9). You may also release the leg by lying on the bed on your abdomen and placing a pillow under your thigh for support as the hip is rotated slightly more anterior. (See Figure 3.14 in Chapter 3.)

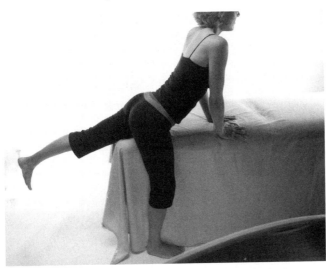

Fig. 19.9. Release position for anterior hip rotation (longer leg)

TEENAGE TELEPHONE TALK (CHAPTER 3) ⫰⫰

➤ Lying on your abdomen (prone), bend your knees so your feet are up in the air. Slowly draw circles in the air with your feet, noting where in the circle there is more ease and comfort. You may pause and rest in any comfortable position for a few moments.

This exercise is named Teenage Telephone Talk because it captures the mood of a relaxed teen, unconsciously self-balancing the pelvis while chatting on the phone (Figure 19.10). This movement exercise helps the sacroiliac joint maintain flexibility. See Chapters 3 and 17 for more releases and movement exercises for the sacroiliac joint.

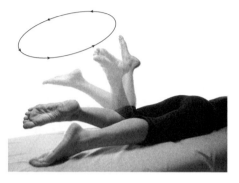

Fig. 19.10. Teenage Telephone Talk: Foot circles help the sacroiliac joint stay flexible

Reestablish the Lumbar Curve with Exercises from Chapter 11

DEVELOP AN AWARENESS OF THE SIT BONES (CHAPTER 11) ⁄⁄⁄⁄⁄⁄⁄⁄⁄⁄⁄⁄⁄⁄⁄⁄⁄⁄⁄⁄⁄⁄

➤ Reeducation of the lumbar curve in the low back begins with an assessment of the sit bones. Check to see if there is even weight distribution on each of the sit bones (Figures 19.11 and 19.12). Uneven weight could be a sign to work with the hip rotation or quadratus lumborum exercises in Chapter 3, or that there is an uneven use pattern in the muscles of the low back. Work with the low back exercises in Chapter 2 and the "Finding the Midpoint of Pelvic Rotation" exercise below (repeated from Chapter 11).

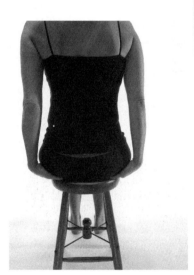

Fig. 19.11. Contact sit bones

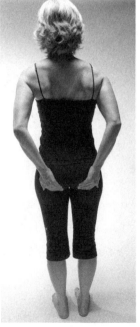

Fig. 19.12. Locate sit bones. Is there even weight on both bones when you sit?

FINDING THE MIDPOINT OF PELVIC ROTATION (CHAPTER 11) ⁗⁗⁗⁗⁗⁗

This movement exercise is another key for working with scoliosis. It helps you to assess and open up balanced movement potential in the hips, pelvis, and lower back for a fuller range of motion. This exercise will reeducate the lumbar curve while building postural strength and flexibility in your lower back. Please refer to Chapter 11 for more information on this exercise and on balancing the spinal curves.

➤ Slowly rotate the pelvis forward, sensing if you are using your muscles evenly on both sides (Figure 19.13). Notice your sit bones as you rotate. Then slowly rotate the pelvis back with the same sensing awareness of your muscles (Figure 19.14). Repeat this rotation sequence five times, cutting a bit off the end each time until you reach a midpoint (Figure 19.15). Once you have found your midpoint, do not try to hold yourself in this posture. Just resume your normal sitting posture or get up and walk around. Practice this exercise a few times daily.

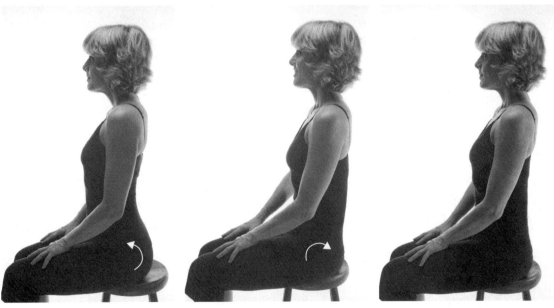

Fig. 19.13. Rotate pelvis forward   Fig. 19.14. Rotate pelvis back   Fig. 19.15. Midpoint

Address the Upper Spine and Rib Cage
with Movement Exercises and Release Positions

- Disc Fluffer and Rotating Disc Fluffer to gain flexibility in the upper spine (from Chapters 10 and 11).

- Assess and combine upper back rotation and lateral-bending preferences (in Chapter 10).

- Releases for ribs and diaphragm (Chapter 12).

MOVEMENT EXERCISE TO REEDUCATE THE CURVE
FOR THE UPPER BACK: DISC FLUFFER (CHAPTER 10) ,,

The following two Disc Fluffer exercises from Chapters 10 and 11 increase flexibility in the upper and mid spine by "fluffing the discs." Try to do these exercises daily as a way to release upper-back fixations and to increase movement in the spine.

➤ Sit with your arms crossed, and let your chin drop forward to your chest. Bring your attention to your upper back, and from there slowly begin a gentle bouncing movement in your upper spine. See if you can sense the bouncing movement at each vertebra level. As you bounce, your head will slowly move toward your lap, but you are not initiating the movement from your neck or head but rather at the spine itself. As you continue to bounce, allow your body to roll forward and your upper back to curl even more. When you have reached a comfortable forward limit, sense the curl of the thoracic area, and then while continuing the gentle bounce, begin to uncurl the spine, slowly bouncing at each vertebra level as you rise from the lower vertebrae (Figures 19.16 to 19.22).

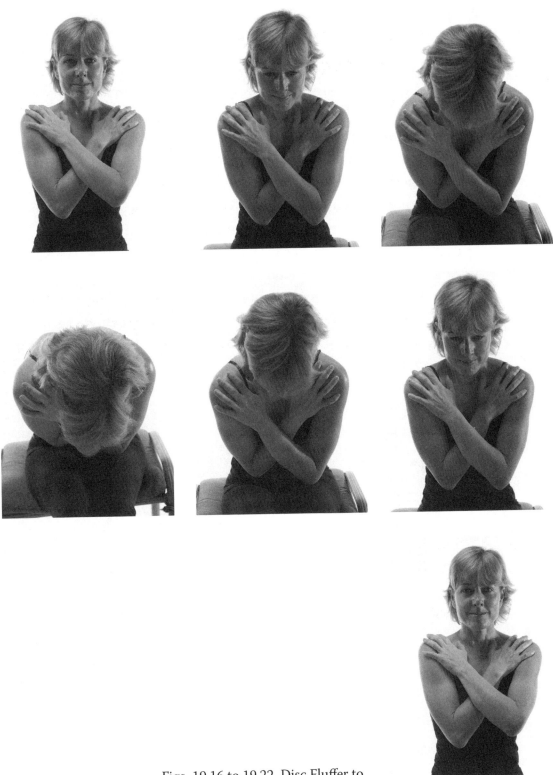

Figs. 19.16 to 19.22. Disc Fluffer to
encourage upper-back flexibility

ROTATING DISC FLUFFER (CHAPTER 11) ///

In this variation of the above exercise you rotate (twist) the spine before beginning the gentle bouncing movement that softly "fluffs" the gelatinous discs that serve as shock absorbers for your spine.

➤ As above, sit with arms crossed over your chest, holding onto the opposite shoulder. Allow your head to roll slightly forward, bringing the spine into a natural posterior curl. Then rotate (twist) to one side, begin the gentle bouncing movement in your upper spine, and allow your body to roll further into a curled position. When you have reached a comfortable forward limit, slowly begin to uncurl the spine, bouncing at each vertebra level as you gradually rise to an upright posture (Figures 19.23 to 19.26).

Rotate your spine to the opposite side and repeat the gentle bouncing on this side as well (Figures 19.27 to 19.30). Pick the most comfortable direction to do first. Stay within your comfort zone and do not do any exercise that causes you pain.

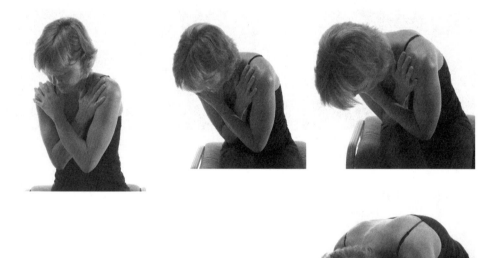

Figs. 19.23 to 19.26. Rotating Disc Fluffer
to encourage upper-back flexibility

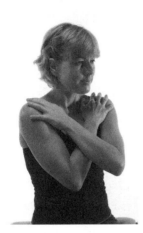
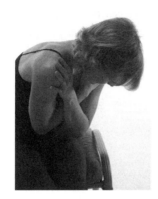
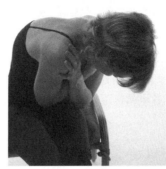
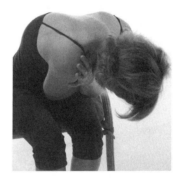

Figs. 19.27 to 19.30. Rotating Disc Fluffer
to encourage upper-back flexibility

SPINAL ROTATION PREFERENCE //

➤ Sitting, rotate your spine first in one direction and let it rebound or bounce back to midline (Figs. 19.31 and 19.32). Then rotate your spine in the other direction (Fig. 19.33) and let it rebound to neutral. Which direction feels most comfortable to you? Sit in the position of your rotation preference for ten to thirty seconds. Repeat this exercise frequently to begin to loosen rotational patterns in the spine.

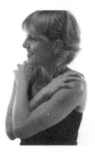 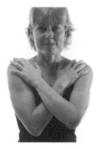 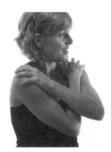

Figs. 19.31 to 19.33. Check for rotation preference

SPINAL SIDE-BEND PREFERENCE //

➤ Sitting, side-bend to the right, slowly bringing your right shoulder toward your right hip. Be careful to keep your head, neck, and upper body in the same plane as the hips, as if between two panes of glass. Note any tension, restriction, or pain as you make the movement. Only move as far as is comfortable. Return to center (Figures 19.34 and 19.35).

Next, laterally bend to the left, bringing your left shoulder toward the left hip with the same considerations (Figure 19.36). Which direction feels more comfortable to you? Sit in the position of your side-bend preference for ten to thirty seconds.

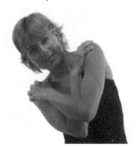 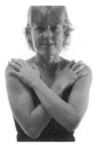 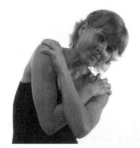

Figs. 19.34 to 19.36. Check side-bend preference

COMBINE ROTATION AND SIDE-BEND PREFERENCE ,,,

➤ Slowly move into a position that combines your rotation preference and your side-bend preference. Explore to see just the right amount of rotation and side-bend that is most comfortable and easy for you. For some the movement may be very slight or subtle. Rest in this position for ten to thirty seconds (Figure 19.37).

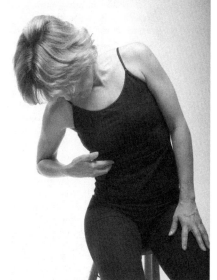

Fig. 19.37. Combining (left) rotation preference with (left) side-bend preference

GENERAL RELEASE POSITIONING FOR THE RIB CAGE ,,,,,,,,,,,,,,,,,,,,,,,,,,,,,,,,,,,,,,,

➤ Sometimes in scoliosis tension patterns are held in the ribs. For tension or tenderness on the side of the rib cage, slowly side-bend (shoulder to hip) and rotate the torso, curving around any tight or tender areas for ten to thirty seconds or until tenderness is relieved (Figure 19.38). You may fine-tune the position by monitoring any tender point with your finger to see when it begins to release.

Move slowly in an exploratory manner to locate the release position. Quicker movements tend to skip past the position of optimal relief.

If general positioning doesn't seem to work, please refer to Chapters 12 and 20 for more rib releases.

Fig. 19.38. Side-bend and curl around sore rib

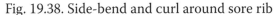

DIAPHRAGM RELEASE (CHAPTER 12)⟋⟋⟋⟋⟋⟋⟋⟋⟋⟋⟋⟋⟋⟋⟋⟋⟋⟋⟋⟋⟋⟋⟋⟋⟋⟋⟋⟋⟋⟋⟋⟋⟋⟋

Often tension in the ribs comes from holding patterns in the diaphragm muscle. This exercise addresses this muscle and also helps to open up flexibility between the lower and upper back.

➤ Lie on your back with a pillow placed under your hips. Bend both knees up and let them fall open to a comfortable relaxed position (Figure 19.39). Allow the legs to move to the most comfortable position for you. Rest in this position for ten minutes.

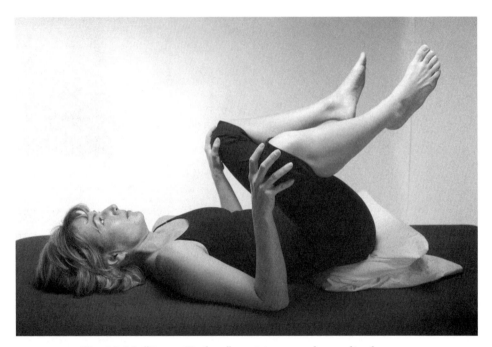

Fig. 19.39. "Roast Turkey" position to release diaphragm.
Allow your legs to move to the most comfortable position for you.

Put It All Together with Balanced Sitting Posture

- Combining Disc Fluffer with Finding your Midpoint (Chapter 11).

- Combine Rotation and Side-Bend Preference to Create a Visually Straight Spine (in this chapter).

- Supporting the Natural Curves While You Sleep—a bedtime towel exercise to maintain flexibility and spinal curves (Chapter 11).

COMBINING DISC FLUFFER WITH FINDING YOUR MIDPOINT (CHAPTER 11) ⫫⫫

This exercise combines the Disc Fluffer and Finding the Midpoint exercises to assist you in establishing a more balanced posture. When this exercise is done well, you will begin to reeducate the lumbar curve to the most functional midpoint, and the upper back to its more natural posterior curve. You should feel more relaxed in your shoulders and more balanced in your spine, with the weight supported by the pelvis.

➤ As in the basic Disc Fluffer exercise, cross your arms over your chest, roll your head forward, and begin a gentle bouncing movement as you allow your thoracic spine to curl forward (Figure 19.40).

Then, with your head down and your thoracic spine rounded, bring awareness to your sit bones. Rotate your pelvis ("tricycle wheels") forward just to the midpoint that you found earlier with this exercise. Be sure you are initiating the movement in your pelvis with awareness of your sit bones and not from your waist or upper body (Figure 19.41).

Once you have arrived at your midpoint with your head down and chin tucked, maintain the curl in the upper spine while slowly allowing your curled upper spine to move directly back until your shoulders are aligned over your hips (Figure 19.42). At this point your chin is still tucked and the upper back maintains a slight posterior curve; your shoulders are aligned over your hips. Now slowly raise your head to upright (Figure 19.43).

Monitor yourself and your sensations carefully, so you don't simply resume your familiar pattern. The most common mistakes in this exercise are initiating movement to the midpoint from the waist or rib level and pulling the shoulders back by straightening the spine and thereby losing the thoracic curve.

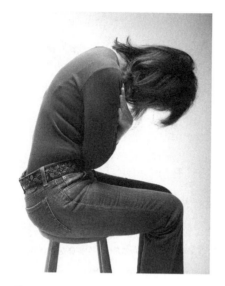

Fig. 19.40. Disc Fluffer

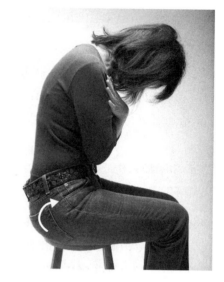

Fig. 19.41. Rotate hips to midpoint

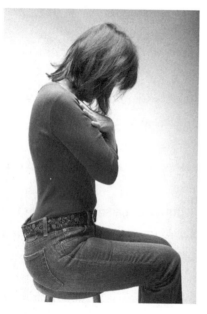

Fig. 19.42. Bring shoulders over hips

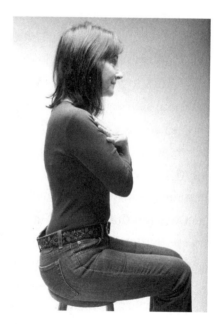

Fig. 19.43. Lift head

COMBINE ROTATION AND SIDE-BEND PREFERENCE TO CREATE A VISUALLY STRAIGHT SPINE ,,

In this exercise you will combine two of the upper-back movement preferences to create a visually aligned spine. This exercise can be subtle, and it helps to have a friend standing behind you to monitor your spine. If you have more than one C curve (sideways curve) in your spine, just pick one curve to work with at a time.

➤ Move very slowly into a position that combines your rotation preference and your side-bend preference (Figure 19.44). Explore to determine just the right amount of rotation and side-bend that is most comfortable and easy for you. With this exercise it is most useful to have a friend monitor your spine for better alignment of the vertebrae as you slowly rotate and side-bend toward your preferences. The combined rotation and side bend may cause the upper back and rib cage to appear twisted or your shoulder or hip to be higher, but have your friend check to see if the spinal vertebrae appear straighter and more in alignment. When you have reached this place of alignment and if you feel comfortable in this position, sit there for only as long as you feel comfort. For some that might mean a few seconds; for others it might be a minute or two.

This can be a potent exercise for the reeducation of the spinal muscles, so it is important that you not overdo it. Overstraining weak muscles that you are attempting to awaken and strengthen will only cause the body to create further tension patterns or resume the familiar holding pattern. If you start to feel tension or discomfort anywhere in your pelvis or spine then let go of the exercise, resume your regular activities, and revisit the exercise again later in the day. You may practice sitting like this a couple of times daily.

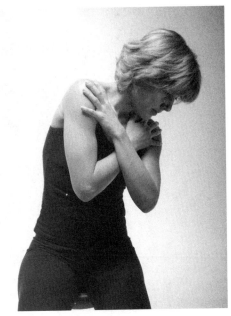

Fig. 19.44. Combining (left) rotation preference with (left) side-bend preference (Chapter 10)

SUPPORTING THE NATURAL CURVES WHILE YOU SLEEP (CHAPTER 11) ,,,,,,,

➤ First prepare the rolled hand towels by folding them in half lengthwise, then folding both sides into the midline, and then rolling them as shown in Chapter 11 (Figures 11.2 to 11.6). Standing, raise the elbows to shoulder height with hands overlapping in front of your face. Rotate the elbows and upper torso to the left as far as is comfortable, and then swing the elbows and upper torso back to the right. Do this rotation exercise about forty times in each direction nightly before bed (Figures 19.45 to 19.48).

Lie with one rolled hand towel under your waist and the other behind your neck for at least twenty minutes (Figure 19.49). If you are comfortable you may fall asleep on them. If after twenty minutes you can't sleep, move into your normal sleeping position. This exercise is useful throughout your reeducation program, as it warms the discs and reminds the body of its movement potential.

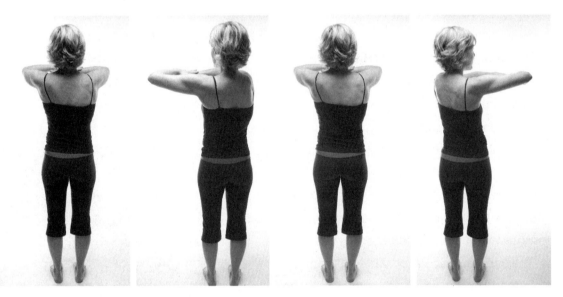

Figs. 19.45 to 19.48. Spinal rotation
to warm discs (Chapter 11)

Fig. 19.49. Lie on rolled towels to
reeducate spinal curves

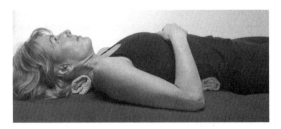

⁓⁓⁓

CHAPTER 20

Repetitive Strain and Carpal Tunnel Syndrome

Repetitive strain and carpal tunnel syndrome are cumulative stress disorders that affect more than one area of the body. Repetitive motions and overuse can cause muscles in the arms and hands to become tight, sore, and tired. Attempting to relieve the strain, the body develops compensatory postures and holding in the shoulders, neck, and back. Unfortunately, these postural misalignments further contribute to the stress.

The nervous system can become locked in a feedback loop as increased muscle contractions attempt to quiet the overstimulation. When these spasms and tensions extend to the upper spine and neck area, an impingement of the nerves to the arms and wrists can result in numbness, weakness, aches, and pain.

Often the person loses all capacity for rest and recuperation because the sympathetic nervous system is on overload, and the parasympathetic nervous system cannot get the deep rest needed to reestablish balance and well-being. The entire body can become locked into patterns of tension, exhaustion, weakness, and pain.

With any cumulative stress disorder—whether fibromyalgia, carpal tunnel, or the cumulative stress that builds up after an injury—quieting the nervous system, relieving the pain, and reestablishing balanced reflexes are the goals. The capacity of this gentle work to effectively meet these goals is illustrated by the story of the original positional release client.

In a paper entitled "Spontaneous release by positioning,"[1] Lawrence Jones, an osteopathic physician, described the frustrating case of a patient with a low back injury that resulted in a chronic 2nd lumbar misalignment and inflamed psoas muscle. The man's condition kept him from standing upright, and the pain and discomfort were so intense that he was unable to sleep, waking with pain every few minutes.

After unsuccessfully treating him for months, Jones devoted an entire session to finding a comfortable position in which the man could rest. Jones moved the man very slowly, passively exploring his range of motion to find a position that would relieve the pain. When an optimal position of comfort was found, even though it was a surprisingly extreme position, the patient relaxed and slept. Jones let him sleep while he left the room to treat another patient. When he returned he found that his patient had increased mobility and a two-thirds reduction of pain. He was able to stand upright for the first time in months, and his structural misalignments had spontaneously corrected.

You may not be able to find one single position that will relieve all the tension in your whole body. Yet, by cultivating your capacity for deep relaxation as you move through the release positions for each of the affected areas, you will be making progress toward your goals of pain relief, quieting the nervous system, and reestablishing balance in the reflexes.

A student in one of my Self-Care courses who suffers with chronic pain became frustrated while trying out release positions in class. She was looking for her whole body to relax and release from one position and became upset that it didn't seem to be working. Even as one area released, pain in other areas distracted her from feeling comfort in that release. I suggested that she just focus on releasing one point at a time and sense the release taking place in that one area. I encouraged her to place her attention on what felt better and not to worry about the places that had not cleared yet. As she focused her attention to each release position, her anxiety diminished along with her pain. She was smiling as she shared with me that with her focus on comfort and relaxation, she discovered that she could self-regulate toward that goal.

Wrists, hands, arms, elbows, shoulders, ribs, neck, spine, and posture are areas affected by carpal tunnel syndrome and repetitive strain injury. I encourage you to work with the releases for each of these areas, one at a time. Points and positions specific to working with pain in the arm, shoulder, and hand are presented below.

With any cumulative pain syndrome, release the lower back, pelvis, and spine as well as working at the site of pain. Bringing balance and alignment to the foundation of the body allows the upper body to rest down more easily. Releasing the 5th lumbar and balancing hip rotations is especially important for fibromyalgia as well as upper-body tension and pain.

Remember, cumulative stress conditions build up over time. With each moment you spend in a release position you are beginning to reeducate, reinforce, and accumulate a new learned sense of ease and relief. Invest the time in yourself to explore for comfort so you can cultivate a condition of cumulative ease.

Anatomy of the Brachial Plexus

There is a network of nerves that originate between the vertebrae of the neck and extend down through the shoulder to the arm and hand (Figure 20.1). This network is called the brachial plexus. Tension or tight contractions of muscles in the neck, shoulder, and arm can impinge on these nerves, causing weakness and pain in the arm, shoulder, and hand.

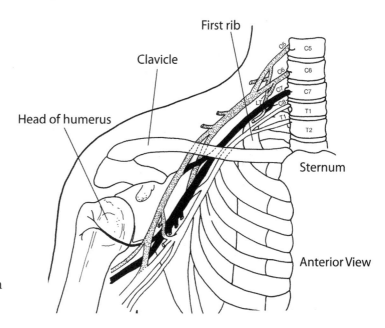

Fig. 20.1. Brachial plexus. Courtesy of *Illustrated Essentials of Musculoskeletal Anatomy,* 4th Edition, by Sieg and Adams (Gainesville, FL: Megabooks, Inc., 1992), www.muscleanatomybook.com

Releasing Nerve Pain in the Shoulder, Arm, Hand, and Fingers

The next three release positions are especially effective for nerve pain in the arms, shoulders, wrists, hands, and fingers. Two of these address tension surrounding the 3rd rib. The importance of addressing the 3rd rib became apparent when I began working with clients with carpal tunnel syndrome. These techniques quiet the nervous system and assist the various muscle tension patterns in the ribs, shoulder, and back to release. As the muscles let go of their tension, pressure diminishes on the nerves of the wrist, arm, and hand. The 3rd rib techniques can also help with lymph drainage, rapid heartbeat (myocarditis), symptoms of asthma, and most interestingly, the release of soft tissues in the foot. I have used the releases for 3rd rib and Parker's Reflex along with the 1st rib, shoulder, wrist, and hand releases to relieve carpal tunnel symptoms and "trigger" spasms in the thumbs and fingers.

For nerve pain that is particularly severe at night, sleep in a side position with your upper (affected) arm at your side or behind you on a pillow. If your arm falls forward, you may be adding compression to the brachial plexus area, irritating the nerves there even further. If you are uncomfortable letting your arm rest behind you, be sure to try the Cross Pull Release for front arm indicator points in Chapter 14.

NERVE PAIN RELEASE USING 3RD RIB POINTS: ROLL THE SHOULDER ,,,,,,,,,,,

Tension around the 3rd rib often results in arm, shoulder, or hand pain (Figure 20.2). Check for tenderness between the 3rd and 4th ribs near the sternum or on the 3rd rib itself where it meets the sternum.

➤ Find the 3rd rib by counting down from the collarbone. The 1st rib is a bony lump just below where the clavicle meets the sternum. Under the 1st rib, feel a space and then just below that space, contact the bone of the 2nd rib. The head of the 2nd rib where it meets the sternum is usually prominent and easy to find. Continue feeling and counting down the spaces and the bones next to the sternum. You may find a tender point on the bone of the

3rd rib or in the space between the 2nd and 3rd or between the 3rd and 4th (Figure 20.3).

Sitting, gently grasp and slowly roll the shoulder toward the front midline of the body. Once in the position you may let go of the shoulder and return to monitoring the release point to sense for softening or pulsing at the point. Hold this relaxed position for twenty to sixty seconds (Figure 20.4).

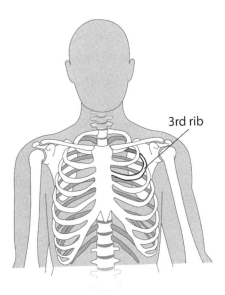

Fig. 20.2. Left 3rd rib

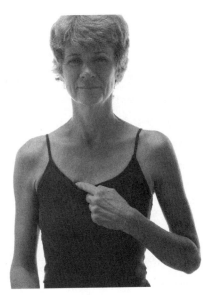

Fig. 20.3. Right 3rd rib point

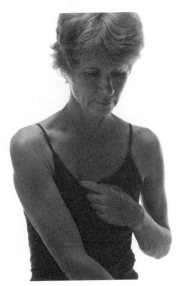

Fig. 20.4. Release position for nerve pain in right arm

ALTERNATE 3RD RIB RELEASE: 3RD RIB COMES HOME ///////////////////////////////

➤ For this exercise you can either sit or you can lie on your opposite side with your affected arm resting at your side or slightly behind you on a pillow. If you are lying down be sure that the affected arm does not fall toward the front of the body.

Using your opposite hand, place the thumb on the tender 3rd rib where it meets the sternum. Place your middle finger on the same rib where it curves up in the armpit. You will know you are in the right place if the rib there feels tender or sore. Once you have found the place, relax your contact to be very light (Figure 20.5).

Sense the shoulder and arm drop slightly as you consciously relax the area. You may sense a slight movement of the rib cage and shoulder as the area relaxes, or you may notice a pulsation, a slight movement, or heat at your contacting fingers. This release can be subtle, and it takes a bit longer. Keep the relaxed contact for a few minutes to ensure a release. I have monitored these points until the whole area around the 3rd rib releases and the points feel completely neutral, which can take up to fifteen or twenty minutes.

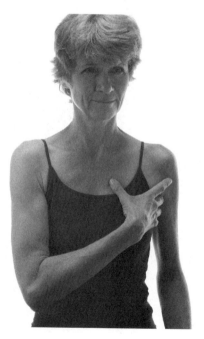

Fig. 20.5. Release for left 3rd rib

RELEASE FOR PARKER'S REFLEX POINT ,,

This point, named after osteopathic physician E. Tracy Parker, is one of the most effective points I have found to release chronic or acute pain in the arm, shoulder, and hand. I use it for arm, shoulder, or hand pain, carpal tunnel and repetitive strain concerns, fibromyalgia, and frozen shoulder conditions. This point is also tender for Dupuytren's contractures,[2] a condition in which the hands develop ropey contractions in the palm and the fingers contract into flexed positions. Use the release below as well as all techniques for the hands and arms and 3rd rib.

The Parker's reflex point is located on the upper lateral (outside) edge of the shoulder blade just below the head of the humerus (upper arm bone). See Figure 20.6.

Though releasing this Parker's reflex point on your own can be difficult, it proves well worth it to enlist a friend's help (Figure 20.7).

➤ Begin by lying face down, head turned to the same side as the tender point. Your friend stands or kneels on the side opposite the tender point, then reaches across your back, grasps your affected elbow, and gently pulls the elbow up and across toward the spine. Fine-tune for comfort or maximum release at the point by bringing the arm slightly down toward the feet or gently up toward the neck while maintaining a slight pull toward the midline of the body. This midline pull creates caving and compression around the point, and the fine-tuning helps to identify just the right direction of pull (Figure 20.8).

Your friend can monitor the point for a pulsating release with the middle finger of his free hand while maintaining the position.

Meanwhile, you relax and allow the shoulder muscles to remain passive as your friend pulls and holds. Your friend should maintain your arm in the most comfortable position for about thirty to sixty seconds.

If pulling the arm back is uncomfortable for you, you may need to release the arm points on the front of the body first (Chapter 14, Cross Pull) or Shoulder Points 1 and 2 in Chapter 13. Then try the Parker's position again with slightly less pull to see if that feels more comfortable.

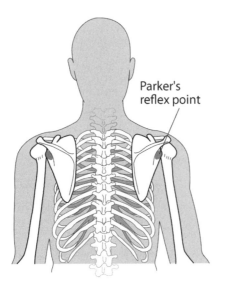

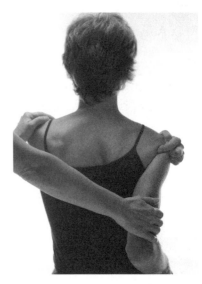

Fig. 20.6. Parker's reflex points

Fig. 20.7. Friend releases
Parker's point

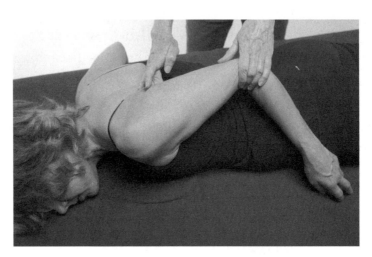

Fig. 20.8. Friend releases Parker's point

※※※

CHAPTER 21

Anxiety, Chronic Fatigue, and Insomnia

Continuous stresses to the body-mind can lead to an overstimulated nervous system that can't find its way back into balance. Chronic pain, nagging worry, and anxiety can prevent the body from getting the rest and recuperation needed for optimal functionality. Ongoing fatigue, lack of energy, inability to concentrate, loss of appetite, and insomnia can all be symptoms of a nervous system that is out of balance.

Even with a chronic condition of nervous system overload, daily attention to releasing Chapman's reflex points in your upper chest can help your body relax and the nervous system to rebalance.

Remember to be patient and hold compassion for yourself. Gradual recognition of your body's self-corrective ability will come as you are able to reduce or clear the tenderness and discomfort at each of these reflex points, one point at a time. As you trust in the process and learn to rest in comfort, your sense of comfort and relaxation will increase and spread to neighboring areas.

Practicing Square Breathing (see the Introduction) also helps you recalibrate your nervous system, and you can do it throughout the day.

RELEASE FOR AN OVERSTIMULATED NERVOUS SYSTEM:
"I SURRENDER"

Tenderness to the touch of the entire upper chest and particularly in the area of the 4th rib can indicate an overstimulated nervous system. Address one point at a time, sensing its release, then moving to the next point and sensing that release (Figure 21.1).

➤ If sitting, gently roll your shoulder and upper body forward to curl around the points (Figure 21.2). Even better, lie down—perhaps with a pillow on your chest—and gently pull the arm of your affected side across your torso, rolling that shoulder toward the sternum, and then let your arm feel supported across the pillow. Allow yourself to surrender to the sensations of comfort and relaxation.

Monitor any sore points you find in your upper chest, particularly at 4th rib. Remember to monitor the tender points with a very light, minimal contact. You may sense a release of heat, slight pulsation, or softening. If the area is particularly charged up you may even feel a subtle buzzing. Continue to lightly monitor the points with a relaxed manner until the entire area feels less tender, less reactive, or neutral.

Relax into the position for as long as you are comfortable, and perhaps drift off for a nap (Figure 21.3).

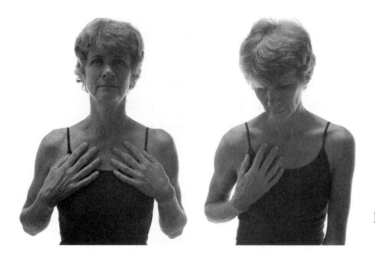

Fig. 21.1. Tender points for overstimulated nervous system

Fig. 21.2. Release position to quiet the nervous system

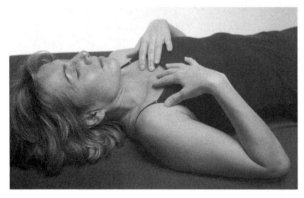

Fig. 21.3. Quiet the nervous system

RELEASE POSITION FOR INSOMNIA INDICATOR POINTS:
DIAL-A-FRIEND,,

By relaxing tension at the insomnia points, even extreme nervousness can be relieved, so you drop off to sleep easily and return to sleep easily if awakened during the night. Releasing these points can ease menopausal insomnia as well.

Like the release for Parker's reflex, insomnia points are best released with the help of your partner or a friend.

The indicator points for insomnia are located all along the top edge of the shoulder blade (Figures 21.4 and 21.5). An additional point can be found on the face of the 4th rib in back, just next to the inner edge of the shoulder blade. To find the 4th rib, count down from the 7th cervical, which is the biggest bump at the top of the spine. The next small bump is the first thoracic and so you would count down each small bump until you get to the 4th and then come lateral to reach the 4th rib (Figure 21.4).

➤ Begin by lying on your stomach, making sure that your neck is comfortable.

Your friend feels for tenderness along the top of the shoulder blade and on the 4th rib and will monitor these tender indicator points.

He or she then places the other hand at the base of your shoulder blade, fitting the bottom corner of your scapula between his/her forefinger and thumb. Gently pushing your shoulder blade toward the top of the shoulder, your friend can feel for softening, pulsing, or relaxing at the indicator points (Figures 21.6 and 21.7).

This position can be held for up to a minute. You may need to release these points only once, or you may need to release them daily for several days in a row. Release the points as close to bedtime as is convenient.

One woman who has a habit of waking in the middle of the night said she could release it by herself by propping her elbow onto a pillow while lying on her side and just holding a gentle contact on the points until they released. The propped elbow shortened the muscles above the border of the scapula and relaxed them, allowing her to return to sleep.

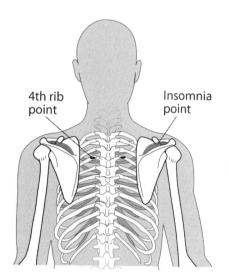

4th rib
point

Insomnia
point

Fig. 21.4. Insomnia points

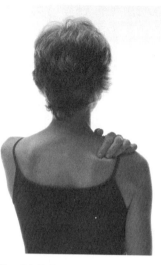

Fig. 21.5. Insomnia points

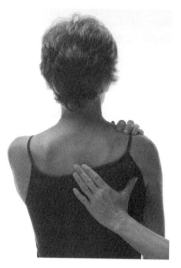

Fig. 21.6. Friend compresses
bottom of scapula toward
points to relieve insomnia

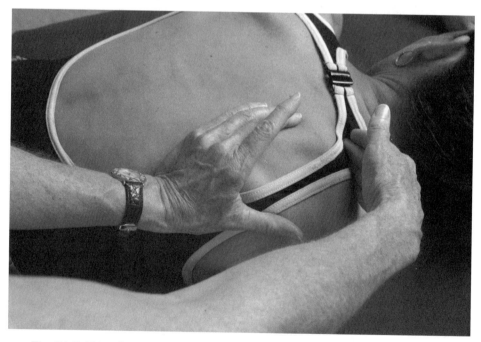

Fig. 21.7. Friend compresses from bottom of scapula toward top border
to release tension points

※※※

Suggested Sequence for Self-Care of Cumulative Stress Disorders

Repetitive Strain, Fibromyalgia, Carpal Tunnel Syndrome, Chronic Fatigue, Anxiety

- Begin with, and revisit frequently, the releases for the low back and pelvis (Chapters 2 and 3). This area is the foundation for good posture and structural well-being. Foundational stability, particularly the 5th lumbar release and the hip release, is essential for relief of fibromyalgia. Remember to do the Abdominal Breathing with the lumbar release (Chapter 2).

- Use the release positions for a rotated hip imbalance and the movement exercises to keep the sacroiliac joint open (Chapter 3).

- Release the upper back, especially in cases of arm, hand, and shoulder pain (Chapter 10).

- Release the 1st rib (Chapter 12), Shoulder Points in Chapter 13, neck in Chapter 15, and ribs in Chapter 12.

- Release the arm points in Chapter 14, with special attention to the two Dial-A-Friend releases: Parker's Reflex Release in Chapter 20, and Insomnia Release in this chapter (21), and both nerve pain releases: Roll the Shoulder and 3rd Rib Comes Home, both in Chapter 20.

- Release the wrist, elbow, and hand (Chapter 14) as needed.

- Practice the postural exercises in Chapter 11 to maintain ease of movement and flexibility.

- Practice the Square Breathing technique (from the Introduction) to calm the nervous system.

GLOSSARY

anterior. Front of the body.

ASIS (Anterior Superior Iliac Spine). Front part of hip bone.

autonomic nervous system. Self-regulating network composed of sympathetic and parasympathetic nerves.

axial. Middle line of the body.

brachial plexus. A network of nerves originating between the vertebrae of the neck, crossing in front of the shoulder, and continuing to various areas of the arm.

carpals. Five long bones of the hand between the finger bones and the wrist bones.

cervical vertebrae. Seven spinal bones making up the neck, extending from base of skull to first thoracic vertebra.

clavicle. Collarbone, extending from the sternum to the top of the scapula.

coccyx. Tailbone.

coracoid process. Small nose-like part of the scapula that extends anterior (forward) to the front of the body. Palpable just medial to the ball of the humerus.

cuboid. Bone on lateral side of foot between 5th metatarsal and heel bone.

cunieforms. Three foot bones connecting to the first, second, and third metatarsals and the cuboid and navicular.

curtsy. A bow with one foot crossed over the other.

diaphragm. Large dome-shaped muscle membrane separating the abdominal area from the lungs and heart (thoracic area).

disc. Gelatinous material between the vertebrae that absorbs shocks and gives the spine flexibility.

discharge. Release.

distal. Away from the center of the body.

elbow. Joint consisting of the lower end of the humerus (upper arm bone) and upper ends of the radius and ulna (lower arm bones).

extend. Straighten or, pertaining to the spine, arch backwards.

flex. Bend.

femur. Bone of the upper leg. Its upper head goes into the hip socket; lower end creates the knee joint.

fibula. Smaller bone on the lateral side of the lower leg that provides support for the tibia.

humerus. Upper arm bone forming the top of the elbow joint at its lower end and part of the shoulder joint at its upper end.

hyoid bone. Small horseshoe-shaped bone in the throat area at the front of the upper neck.

hyper-reflexive. Overly responsive reflex activity.

ilium (ilia, pl.). Hip bone(s). The two disc-shaped bones on either side of the sacrum that form part of the pelvis.

indicator points. Points on the body surface that correlate to certain parts of the internal body, indicating which position to use for the release.

inferior. Toward the lower part of the body.

insomnia. Inability to fall asleep or to get enough sleep.

intercostal muscles. Situated between and connecting adjacent ribs.

interosseous membrane. Tissue between the two lower arm bones or between the two lower leg bones.

ischium (ischia, pl.). Sit bone(s) of the pelvis, at bottom of buttock.

isometric. Muscle stays the same length during resisted attempted movement.

isotonic. Resistance stays the same as muscle gradually lengthens during resisted attempted movement.

lateral. Toward the side of the body.

lateral flexion. Bending to the side of the body.

ligament. Fibrous tissue that connects bones or cartilage at a joint.

lumbar vertebrae. Five large bones of the lower spine from the waist to the top of the hips.

5th lumbar. Lowest lower-back vertebra.

malleolus. Part of the ankle formed by the wider parts of the tibia and fibula.

metacarpals. Cluster of seven small bones at the wrist.

metatarsals. Five long bones in the foot that attach to the toe bones.

motor. Movement.

neurasthenia. Chronic abnormal fatigue from nervous system overload.

neuromuscular. Relationship between nerves and muscles.

occiput. Base of the skull where it meets the 1st cervical (top neck bone).

palpation/palpate. Hand contact with the body, with the focus on sensing the structure beneath the surface.

parasympathetic. System of nerves from the brain and sacral area that innervate the heart, viscera, and glands of the head and neck for the conservation and restoration of the body's energy resources.

patella. Kneecap. A bone that "floats" in front of the knee joint, held in place by numerous ligaments.

peripheral. Away from the center of the body.

phalanges. Toe bones and finger bones.

plantar fasciitis. Inflammation of the fascia of the sole of the foot.

posterior. Back of the body.

prone. Lying face down.

proprioception. System of nerves located in joints, muscles, tendons, and in the labyrinth of the ear, responsible for coordinated movements and our kinesthetic awareness.

proximal. Nearer the center of the body.

PSIS (Posterior Superior Iliac Spine). The spine of the posterior hip.

psoas *(pronounced so-as).* Deep-lying muscle that connects to the front of the spine and attaches to the inside of the thighbone at the lesser trocanter of the femur.

pubic bone. Lower anterior bone of the pelvis.

quadratus lumborum. Deep-lying muscle of the low back that connects the top of the hip bone to the lumbar vertebrae.

radius. Lower arm bone on the thumb side of the arm, extending up to the elbow.

ramus. Part of the pubic bone that branches to connect with a branching part of the ischium (sit bone); found along the inside of the leg.

reflexes *(verb).* Response of a nerve center to a stimulus.

sacroiliac joint. Where sacrum and ilium meet to make a joint.

sacrum. Triangle-shaped bone at the base of the spine; joins to a hip bone on either side and forms part of the pelvis.

scapula. Triangle-shaped bone at the sides of the upper back next to each arm and forming part of the shoulder.

sciatic nerve *(pronounced sigh-attic).* Extends from the sacrum down the back of the leg.

sensory. Sensation.

superior. Toward the top of the body.

sympathetic nervous system. Nerves originating in the thoracic and upper lumbar area that stimulate the use of stored energy to involuntary muscles and glands, most notable in the fight-or-flight response.

talus. Ankle bone that connects the tibia to the foot.

tendon. Strong fibrous tissue that binds muscle to the bone.

thoracic vertebrae. Twelve spinal bones extending from the neck area to behind the waist; each thoracic vertebra has a rib attached to each side.

tibia. Primary weight-bearing bone of the lower leg.

ulna. Lower arm bone on the little-finger side of the arm, extending up to the elbow.

BIBLIOGRAPHY

Alexander, Gerda. 1981. *Eutony: The Holistic Discovery of the Total Person.* New York: Felix Morrow.

Calais Germain, Blandine. 2007. *Anatomy of Movement.* Seattle: Eastland Press.

Deig, D. 2006. *Positional Release Technique.* Indianapolis: Somatic Publications.

Kain, K.L., with Berns, J. 1997. *Ortho-Bionomy: A Practical Manual.* Berkeley, CA: North Atlantic Books.

Moffitt, P. 2008. *Dancing With Life.* New York: Rodale.

Owens, C. 2002. *An Endocrine Interpretation of Chapman's Reflexes.* Indianapolis: American Academy of Osteopathy.

Sarno, J. 1991. *Healing Back Pain: The Mind-Body Connection.* New York: Warner Books.

Seig, K., and Adams, S. 2002. *Illustrated Essentials of Musculoskeletal Anatomy.* Gainesville, FL: Megabooks.

Thie, J., and Thie, M. 2005. *Touch for Health.* Camarillo, CA: DeVorss & Company.

NOTES

Chapter 2: Low Back

1. A book entitled *Healing Back Pain: The Mind-Body Connection* by Dr. John Sarno allegedly helps 80% of those who read it. I have recommended it to many of my clients, who later call me in surprise and astonishment that they have experienced pain relief from the understandings gleaned from the book. You may want to read it and see for yourself.

2. Notes from a Mindful Movement class taught by Phillip Moffitt, Vipassana meditation teacher and author of *Dancing with Life*.

Chapter 3: Pelvis: Sacrum, Hips, Sacroiliac Joint, and Tailbone

1. This condition was named the "pelvic thyroid syndrome" by osteopath Charles Owens in the 1930s and is described in *An Endocrine Interpretation of Chapman's Reflexes.*

   The work of osteopath Frank Chapman in the 1930s brought to light a system of nerve reflexes that demonstrate the relationship between structure and organ function. Many of these neuro-reflex points for the organs are located where the ribs meet the sternum or in the back where the ribs meet the thoracic spine. Releasing these tender points helps to rebalance lymph flow and optimize health. See Chapter 12 on the rib (the section entitled "Breastbone") for how to release them, and Chapter 20 for Parker's reflex and 3rd rib releases for nerve pain in the arm and hand.

2. Charles Owens, DO, *An Endocrine Interpretation of Chapman's Reflexes* (see above).

Chapter 4: Alignment of Hips, Legs, Knees, and Feet

1. Gerda Alexander developed a method she named "Eutony," meaning "well tone." She directed a school in Copenhagen where she worked with musicians, dancers, and "hopeless cases" referred to her by the local hospitals. Gerda was in her eighties when she came to teach in

the San Francisco Bay Area, and I feel so fortunate to have had the opportunity to study with her. Her gentle, inner-focused approach to self-care has influenced my work in so many ways.

Chapter 10: Upper and Mid Back: Thoracic Spine

1. See Note 2, Chapter 2.
2. See Note 1, Chapter 4.

Chapter 11: Spinal Integrity

1. The mitral valve is in the heart and controls blood flow from the left atrium to the left ventricle.
2. Quoted from a video taken by Baelaey Callister in a class taught by Arthur Lincoln Pauls in 1987. The video consists of combined footage from several different classes, with the quoted part from a class in Contra Costa, California.
3. *Touch for Health* by John Thie, DC, compiles practical user-friendly information about acupressure, nutrition, and balanced muscle strength through kinesiology.

Chapter 12: Ribs

1. See Note 1, Chapter 3, in regard to Chapman's work relating reflex points to the body's structure, function, and endocrine system.

Chapter 14: Arms, Elbows, Wrists, and Hands

1. Dupuytren's contractures consist of a thickening of the fibrous tissues in the palm of the hand. The tightening of the tissue can draw the finger(s) toward the palm.

Chapter 15: Neck

1. Eutony means "well tone," a term coined by Gerda Alexander for the subtle awareness and self-healing work she developed in Denmark in the twentieth century. See Chapter 10, Note 2, above.

Chapter 16: Head, Face, Eyes, Ears, and Jaw

1. Hexagram 27 I / The Corners of the Mouth (Providing Nourishment). *I Ching,* translated from Chinese into German by Richard Wilhelm and rendered into English by Cary F. Baynes (Princeton, New Jersey: Princeton University Press).

2. Reflex is a spontaneous response occurring automatically from one part of the body to another as a result of the nervous system's reaction to a stimulus.

Chapter 20: Repetitive Strain and Carpal Tunnel Syndrome

1. L.H. Jones, "Spontaneous Release by Positioning," *D.O.* 4 (1964): pp. 109–116.

2. Dupuytren's contractures consist of a thickening of the fibrous tissues in the palm of the hand. The tightening of the tissue can draw the finger(s) toward the palm, resulting in the inability to straighten the finger(s).

INDEX

About the Author

Since 1978 Luann Overmyer has worked with thousands of people in pain in her Ortho-Bionomy private practice. She teaches thirty Ortho-Bionomy seminars per year, mentors students and instructors, presents at conferences, and writes for newsletters in the United States, Australia, and New Zealand.

She is a registered advanced instructor of Ortho-Bionomy, a licensed massage therapist in Florida, and a Continuing Education provider in Florida and nationally, certified through the National Certification Board for Therapeutic Massage and Bodywork (NCBTMB).

After living three decades near San Francisco and raising her family there, Luann Overmyer currently divides her time among her residence in Fort Pierce, Florida; the San Francisco Bay Area; and Australia.